Lean Life

Lean Life

Get Lean.
Stay Lean.
For Life.

DR. MO

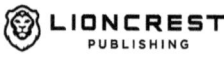

Copyright © 2025 Dr. Mohamed Abdel-Reheim
All rights reserved.

Lean Life
Get Lean. Stay Lean. For Life.

First Edition

ISBN 978-1-5445-4938-5 *Paperback*
       978-1-5445-4937-8 *Ebook*

To Fay,

Because if God wanted me to climb rocks, he would have made me a donkey.

And to everyone who's ever struggled with accepting their own bodies.

Contents

Introduction	1
1. It's Not the Bananas. It's Not the Tuna.	9
2. Saved from the Stinking Chicken	23
3. Eat What You Want—Even Pop-Tarts	55
4. Intermittent Fasting	73
5. Reverse Pyramid Weight Training: Spend Less Time with Sociopaths!	83
6. Lean Life	93

Introduction

I'M AN EGYPTIAN TEXAN, ex-comedian/MD born in Saudi Arabia. Got all that? I moved to Temple, Texas, when I was three years old and don't remember much from Saudi Arabia, except getting my cornea scratched by a cat. But that's another story for another time. Both of my parents are naturalized American citizens from Egypt. My dad was an oceanographer who taught at Texas A&M University—and actually worked with Jacques Cousteau back in the day. My mom is a pathologist. My two older sisters also went to medical school and are doctors.

In other words, medicine is a family thing for me and also a cultural thing. In Egyptian culture, if you're not an engineer, doctor, lawyer, or other highly educated professional, you're basically considered an embarrassment to the family. In the hierarchy of academia, doctor ranks number one.

I went to medical school in Cairo, and while studying there,

I started performing stand-up comedy with other Egyptian American and Egyptian Canadian comedians. In 2009, a group of us got together and put on the first English-language comedy show in Egypt, called Shut Up and Laugh. We attracted nearly a thousand people in the audience. It was an amazing night. Later, I began performing in other countries—in the Middle East and Europe and now in the United States. After earning my medical degree in December 2013, I completed my student internship in Cairo and across the United States, and once my training was complete, I remained in the central Texas area, where I've lived ever since.

I'm telling you all of this so you can understand a little about who I am. But that's not why I've written this book. My experience in Cairo changed my life in another important way. Besides being the place where I got my start in medicine and comedy, it's also where, through several years of research and even more trial and error, I created the Lean Life plan. Through this book, I'm passing my knowledge down to you.

Maybe it's the physician in me, but I feel like I have a responsibility to take an active role in curbing the obesity problem that has arisen not only in our country but also across the globe. By 2030, roughly one-third of the world's population is going to be obese. It's more of a drain on our health-care system than alcoholism and smoking combined, at a cost of $2 trillion a year. Being healthy and in shape is more than about getting ripped and having six-pack abs. It's about knowing moderation and learning beneficial habits.

Nothing makes me happier than to change people's lives for the better when it comes to improving their conditioning and helping them lose weight. One time, during a rotation at a private clinic in Atlanta, I worked closely with an obese patient to plot out an eating and exercise plan and made sure he downloaded MyFitnessPal into his phone before he left the clinic.

INTRODUCTION

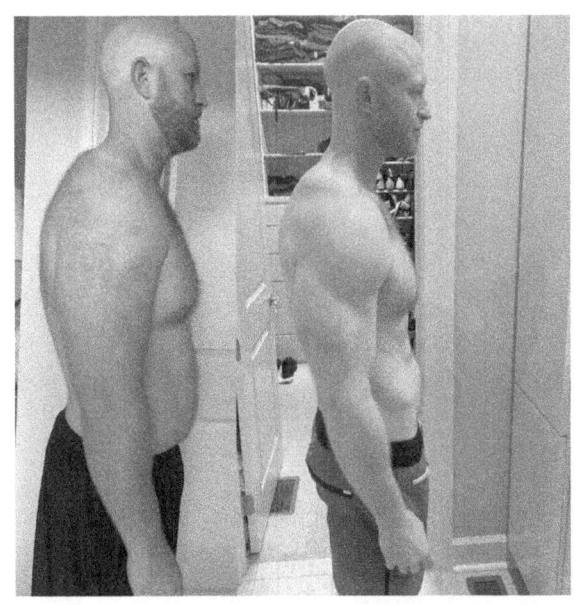

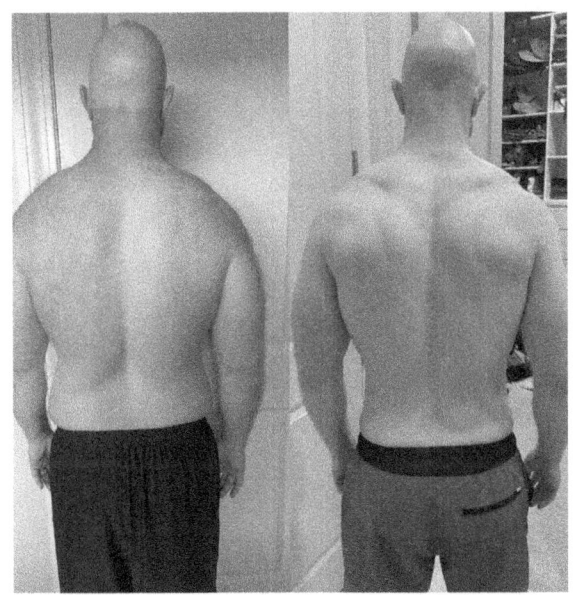

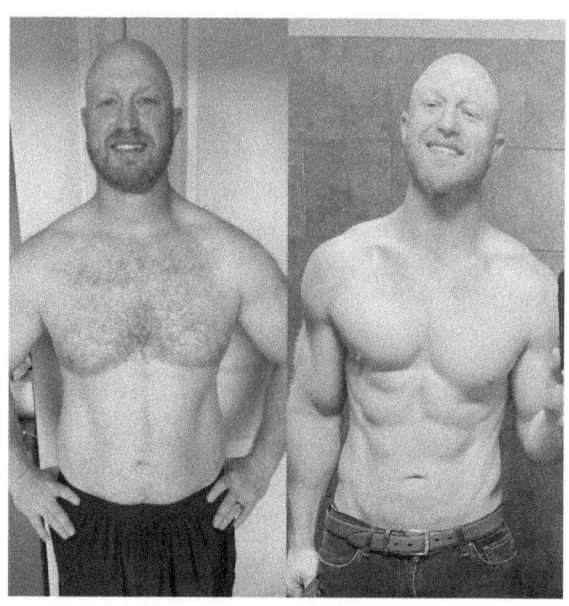

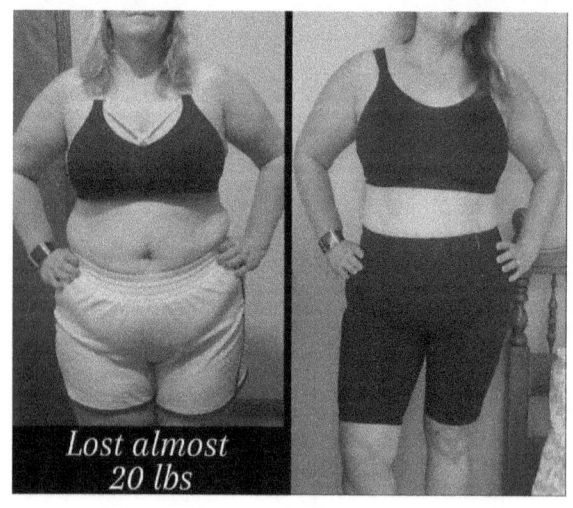

Lost almost 20 lbs

INTRODUCTION

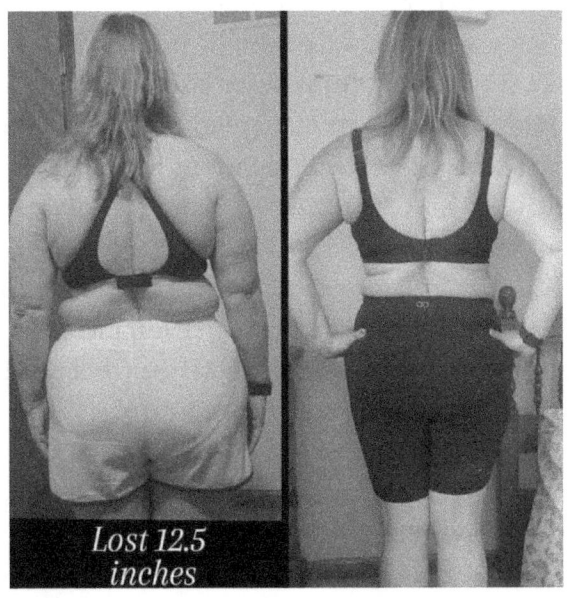

Lost 12.5 inches

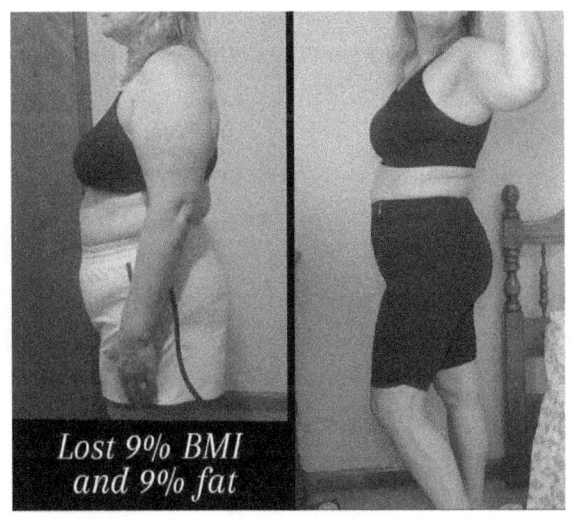

Lost 9% BMI and 9% fat

A few weeks later, I saw him at a restaurant. He said, "Dr. Mo! I've lost ten pounds since the last time I saw you."

It was a very touching experience knowing that I had given him the tools to manage his eating and exercise in a very practical way. It was one of the inspirations that led me to focus my expertise on nutrition and conditioning and to inevitably writing this book.

The Lean Life plan marries three strategies: Flexible Dieting (IIFYM), Intermittent Fasting, and weight training. I'll explain all three in great detail later, but in short, they're aimed at giving you maximum fitness with minimum effort. Yes, you're reading that right: maximum fitness, minimum effort.

I know you've heard sales pitches like this before. But this one is no bullshit. In fact, it's the anti-bullshit. I've been a gym rat since high school, but for the longest time, I've worked out—and dieted—the wrong way, like so many millions of other people. My mistake was believing the garbage that the fitness industry constantly tries to peddle. I didn't realize at the time that they don't really care about your health. They just want you to buy their stupid powders, shakes, pills, or any other instant quick-fix product. Their plans are always complicated and time consuming.

But normal people don't have enough time in the day to spend on elaborate workout routines that show only small benefits. So my aim is to maximize your efficiency in the gym. Get in and get out, get what you need, reap the benefits, and get on with your life. The same concept applies to nutrition and eating. My plan gives you flexibility so you're not wasting time preparing special meal plans, or carrying food in Tupperware containers wherever you go.

I'm not offering some glittery magical treatment for whatever

INTRODUCTION

may ail you. I'm not trying to change you—or even saying that I can. I'm just passing along the knowledge and, more importantly, the perspective, I've gained through my research, experience, and medical background. I'm just trying to tell you that less is more in the long run.

Much of what you read here builds upon concepts pioneered by people such as the self-proclaimed Khan of Intermittent Fasting, Martin Berkhan; conditioning and nutrition badass, and evidence-based researchers Alan Aragon, Eric Helms, and Brad Schoenfeld; revolutionary fitness and workout rebel, and flexible dieting guru Kane Sumabat; and others who I'll be mentioning later. The difference is that I've incorporated my own experiences, research, and medical background with portions of these ideas to give you non-bullshit, science- and evidence-based protocols that fit into one whole-body system that gives great results.

Most of what the people I mention here teach is available online; they have a strong online presence and community. I suggest you check them out. I have a longer list of experts who I have benefited from personally, and whom I suggest you follow, at the end of the book. My hope here is to cut your learning curve and provide a kind of tool by giving you a cross-section of my own personal struggles and insights as an example and allowing you to pick and choose information and advice as you see fit. Or to ignore it altogether and continue to follow "bro" science that you pick up at the gym, or late-night infomercials, or in fitness magazines funded largely by supplement companies.

I hope the Lean Life plan will benefit your life the way it has mine by giving you freedom and flexibility toward your quest to bettering your personal health. Since I began incorporating these tools in my life a few years ago, I've cut my body fat percentage by 50 percent, increased the maximum weight I lift by

50 percent, and improved my emotional state by 100 percent. I'll be throwing a lot of numbers at you, but 50-50-100 is the magic one. If I can get you close to that, we both win. No bullshit.

It's Not the Bananas.
It's Not the Tuna.

If we could give every individual the right amount of nourishment and exercise, not too little and not too much, we would have found the safest way to health.
—Hippocrates

THINK OF ALL OF THE LIES that the fitness industry in America tries to sell you just to make a profit. Then imagine how bad it is in a developing country. This is what I learned firsthand when I went to Egypt in 2007 for medical school.

Basically, fitness instructors in the Middle East are just regular dudes who take a bunch of steroids, get really ripped, and then spend most of their time denying any steroid use. They'll say, "Oh, I just did these exercises and then ate bananas and tuna." Right. Bananas and tuna. That's the popular line or, more accurately, the Untold Truth.

Almost everyone over there knows what the real secret formula is: steroids. And they're very, very popular among gym rats in that part of the world. Egypt has a huge machismo culture, and bodybuilders are big celebrities among their countrymen. I sometimes used to work out at a few different big commercial gyms, and I'd often see pop stars and even Egyptian Mr. Universe competitors working out. It was all very impressive. Then I'd walk into the locker room and see syringes in the garbage can. The temptation to take them was hard to resist.

In the fitness industry, a lot of professional athletes may misguide the public into thinking their crazy physiques are attainable because they claim they follow a natural approach and falsely deny that they use a crazy amount of performance-enhancing drugs. Even worse are the insta-fitness celebrities who flaunt their surgically enhanced derrieres and then try to sell you some magical "tea" that is going to melt the fat away. What they do with their own bodies is, frankly, their own business. They work very hard to be as successful as they are in the professional realm. But they're being reckless by misleading average people into thinking they can attain the same results without the help of steroids or plastic surgery.

When I discovered this reality, I started following the natural bodybuilding community, which has skyrocketed in recent years because of social media. These are the people who you should look to as role models because they provide programs for people with a normal hormonal profile and unaltered biological body parts, not people with thousands of milligrams of testosterone in their bodies or silicone balloons.

There's this inside joke I used to share with a lifting buddy, who was also one of my medical school classmates. It was about this really popular Egyptian professional bodybuilder who competed in Mr. Universe in the early 2000s. We saw him every once in a while working out at one of the gyms where we went. It was very obvious to everyone that he took ridiculous amounts of juice.

One time I turned on the TV and saw him on a kids' TV show, of all places. He said straight into the camera, "Kids,

IT'S NOT THE BANANAS. IT'S NOT THE TUNA.

don't ever take steroids. Don't do that. You need to go big and strong like me."

Then he used the line "All you need is tuna and bananas."

The guy weighs 280 pounds, he's six foot two, all bulging muscle, and he's using the tuna and bananas line. I figured he was sending out two messages. The first was truly to kids, telling them not to take steroids. As a public figure, it's his responsibility to take into consideration that kids look up to him. The second was a kind of nudge and a wink to grown-ups who know that tuna and bananas will never get them that fucking big. I don't care where on the planet the tuna and bananas are coming from. It was almost an enticement to do steroids. After that, whenever my lifting buddy and I saw someone who was clearly taking performance-enhancing drugs, we'd just say the words "bananas and tuna!"

For my first couple years of medical school, as I lived within the crazy juice culture in Egypt, I resisted the temptation of steroids, even as I watched some of my med school classmates get into them. Their bodies would transform. They'd suddenly get massive and fat-free—all 220 pounds of lean muscle mass. I never knew who was on performance-enhancing drugs and who was not.

I was at a loss to find an honest and truthful weight-training program from the gym and community there. I asked some of my buddies and they'd say, "I just lift and take a vitamin. It's just science." And in my mind I'd be thinking, *Shut the fuck up. I'm not an idiot.* It was just another version of the Untold Truth.

I do have to say, though, that part of me was jealous of them. At that time, I worked out pretty regularly at a weight hall—a kind of underground gym—near where I lived. It was a hardcore, old-school place with sand floors that had just weights in it—no machines or anything. No women were allowed either. Most gyms in Egypt are gender-segregated like that.

But as hard as I worked out, using the throwback 1970s classic bodybuilding splits, or "bro" splits, I didn't experience any great results. I wasn't as lean as I knew I could be, and I wasn't as strong either. My whole workout routine was time consuming and ineffective overall, and my nutrition regime was lacking. I began wanting to find a chemical solution and allowed the gym rats there to influence my decisions. Around 2010, I decided to pay a visit to a man I'll call Dr. Juice. Through him, I gave in to the temptation of the tuna and bananas, and made the biggest mistake of my life.

Dr. Juice is an interesting character—a dentist and all-around sociopath. He worked out at my weight hall sometimes. He stood about six foot two, had blue eyes, wore designer clothes that fit him perfectly, and was really, really jacked. Everyone, including me, figured he knew a lot about using steroids safely because of his profession and education.

So we were willing to believe what he was selling, despite the fact that he was selling harmful nonsense. He'd tell anyone, even fifteen-year-old kids, "You're wasting your time at the gym if you don't take juice." Yeah, he was literally Dr. Evil.

I should point out that steroids in Egypt are legal. You can buy them from a pharmacy and even most gyms. Technically, what Dr. Juice was doing wasn't wrong, but the way he was doing it was unethical. He was discouraging a lot of young kids from having the patience, discipline, and dedication to gain muscle mass naturally simply because it's a slower process. To a certain extent, he was saying that it's significantly harder to gain a lot of muscle mass after a year or two of working out, hence people in this boat need to use performance-enhancing drugs to defy this natural physiological ceiling.

Worse yet, he was pretending that he was using science

behind the steroids. He'd say things like "There are seventeen carbons in this," or "This is a short ester, this is a long ester," and everyone believed him because he used big words and there truly is a lot of science behind these chemicals.

He'd tell you not to go anywhere else, like the drug store, to get steroids, claiming that what's on the shelves is fake. Since the drugs were legal, Dr. Juice was such a slick salesman, and I was discouraged about my workouts and jealous of my med school classmates, I decided to meet with him about trying them out. The meeting was at a coffee shop near the gym, and my lifting buddy joined me.

As soon as we sat down with him, he pulled out a piece of paper. On it he wrote the doses we were supposed to take and then handed us some vials of testosterone. He told us we could get the syringes from the supermarket or pharmacy over the counter.

Note to reader: Anytime someone begins a sentence with "And you can buy syringes," walk away. Quickly. We didn't, though. Instead, we followed his instructions. And honestly, it was great—at first.

There's a reason why 80 percent of the people who have used or abused steroids are gym rats. They're not professional athletes, just regular dudes. It's because your strength goes up almost right away, and you don't care about the side effects. You start looking better and people notice you. It's addictive, but it's a big psychological Catch-22. You never believe you're big enough, and you use the image in the mirror to validate yourself. People often get into steroids because they have self-image issues. They lack self-confidence, so they turn to chemical enhancements. They think if they get huge they'll feel better about themselves, but it's like an addiction: too much is never enough.

Steroids tap so deeply into your self-image that it's scary. You start taking them, and then you keep wanting more and more because the minute you stop, you're not as strong, you're not as in shape as you were, you're not as big, you don't think you're as good looking. You don't care what ravages it does to your body, psyche, or emotional control.

After a couple of weeks, I could casually do sets of dumbbell bench presses with 110- and 120-pound dumbbells, which were much heavier weights than I'd ever done before. It was easy to start rationalize what I was doing. I thought, *If so many people are doing other drugs—like drinking, smoking, or whatever—why can't I do one that at least makes me look better?*

But there's a pattern with steroids among people who aren't professional bodybuilders and don't follow a clinically tested and refined regimen. They get in great shape, finish their cycle with the drugs after six or eight weeks, leave the gym for a couple of months, and then eventually come back looking and feeling like crap.

There are nasty side effects too. You start to act strange. You're mean. You're really aggressive. I saw friends just get really batshit crazy from steroid use. Everything for them just revolved around their own self-image and taking juice. That was their whole life.

It affected me too. I went bonkers. I became socially isolated. I became mean. I had a falling out with some of my comedian friends. People began to notice changes in my behavior, especially my family. Once, when my parents and sisters came for a visit to Cairo—something they did once a year—my mom found some of my syringes. I was embarrassed and ashamed—like I was a middle school kid hiding weed—and she thought I was doing something way more serious than steroids, like heroin.

IT'S NOT THE BANANAS. IT'S NOT THE TUNA.

So my family stepped in and held a kind of intervention for me. It was at a time that I wanted to stop on my own. I didn't like the wild swings that steroids sent my body and personality through. The drugs were expensive and reckless, and I had started to realize that they were only going to drag me deeper and deeper into a bottomless hole. The saying goes that doing the same thing over and over again is the definition of insanity. That's how I felt about starting another steroid cycle. Still, I couldn't break free.

Shortly after this, though, the democratic revolution in Egypt occurred. It was January, in 2011. My sister happened to be visiting as millions of protestors marched on Cairo, calling for the removal of President Hosni Mubarak from power. The city became paralyzed. There was a military curfew, the American embassy closed, Internet access was shut down, and even electricity was cut off for a while. Clashes broke out, and people started looting some parts of the city. The airport closed, so we couldn't get out. Meanwhile, I was in mid-cycle on steroids, and that was all I could think about.

There we were, my sister and I, stuck in the capital city of a developing country as a historic, and unpredictable, revolution was catching fire on the streets. And guess what my biggest concern was: getting my next fix, going to the gym, and working out—not safety for my sister, not "freedom for the people," or anything like that. It was crazy. The thought did cross my mind that my priorities were completely screwed up. But my physical urges were stronger than my willpower and the thought process to stop. I was so obsessed with hitting the weights that my buddy and I broke the military curfew to work out. We weren't allowed on the streets after 8:00 p.m., but we still made it our mission to get to the gym. There were tanks on the street, but we didn't care. We were seriously willing to risk being arrested on the spot. That's how crazed I got.

Eventually, the airport opened, and we were able to get tickets back to Texas. The flight included an overnight layover in Frankfort, Germany, which gave me several hours of free time. I found the first gym possible, drank a protein shake, and lifted weights because I didn't want to lose my muscle mass. In the locker room afterward, I thought to myself, *What the fuck is going on? We're literally fleeing a revolution and all I care about is seeing myself in the mirror!* But still, I didn't stop wanting to juice.

Of course, I didn't bring steroids home with me. Even though they're legal and easy to get in Egypt, I would have been committing a felony by carrying them into America. Luckily, I'm not that stupid. So shortly after I got to Texas, feeling the withdrawal from the steroids, I got desperate with worry over losing my "gainz" and my muscle disappearing. It was like I was on crack.

I went to a local gym near my parents' home and asked some meatheads there how to get some steroids. They told me they buy the drugs online from China and get the syringes from a feed store. These guys were complete country farm boys—remember that my hometown is a small town in Texas—and they were shooting themselves with needles made for cattle! That was a bridge too far for me. At that point, I decided to quit juicing altogether, and my short, unsuccessful career as a roid head was over.

I wish I could say that this was the bright beginning of my turnaround toward the much happier, healthier life I live today based on the Lean Life principles. But it wasn't. I kept riding the yo-yo up and down, but mostly further downward for quite a while. When Mubarak was deposed and the protests quieted down, I returned to Cairo, continued with medical school, and

IT'S NOT THE BANANAS. IT'S NOT THE TUNA.

over the course of the next year sank into a deep funk. I gained weight and became socially isolated. I didn't talk to anybody outside of my classes.

In my free time between studies, I became the Binge Watching King. Ask me any question about *Dexter* from any of the show's eight seasons, and I'll answer it. Hey, what better pick-me-up is there than a TV series about a serial killer? I watched Drake music videos nonstop, too, and in my own little irrational world, I wanted to be just like Drizzy. I felt alone in Egypt, with no mentors and no friends whom I thought I could trust. My personal life, including dating, was out. I felt that the only reason that I had value to women when I was juicing was because I had muscles, and that had gone to shit.

I was trapped in a downward spiral. It's actually a very common and powerful side effect of getting off steroids. While you're taking testosterone, your body senses the extra hormones in your system and essentially shuts off its own testosterone production. It doesn't have a job to do anymore. But when you stop taking the drugs, your body doesn't turn the production back on like a light switch. It takes time to get the ignition fired and then back into gear again to ramp up production. In the meantime, your testosterone levels plummet, and you end up feeling pretty shitty.

The resulting funk can feel so profound that it drives people to get back on steroids instead of riding it out. It's like a simple roller-coaster effect. As high into euphoria as steroids send your body, your emotions plummet into an equally deep abyss when you go off cycle. The longer and heavier you get into the drugs, the worse the imbalance can be when you get off. I'm happy my experimentation was very limited. The most important thing I learned was that you need to have a sustainable lifelong approach, not a roller-coaster ride that you get from chemical alternatives.

As I rode out the roller coaster, I turned to Instagram. I needed to find some way to better myself—to get in shape, to lead a healthier lifestyle. Social media was an easy, instant source of information that was right there in my hand, with pictures I could easily see and understand. Each one is worth a thousand words, right?

It didn't take long before a universe of fitness communities opened up to me—all connected by hashtags. I found people sharing sensible information about health and nutrition, and they were showing concrete results through pictures. No tuna and bananas!

Through my browsing, a handful of hashtags kept catching my eye: #FlexibleDieting, #Natty, #NaturalBodybuilding, #MFP (myfitnesspal), #PowerLifting, and especially #IIFYM, which stands for "If It Fits Your Macros." This last one really grabbed my attention. People would post images of themselves eating Pop-Tarts and use the IIFYM hashtag. I thought to myself, *What's this term macros? And why the fuck are these really in-shape people eating Pop-Tarts?* Then I did some more digging.

Through my research, I discovered that "macro" is short for macronutrient—the umbrella term for the three categories of the foods we eat: fat, carbohydrates, and proteins. Counting macros is like taking calorie counting to the next level. It's a way to transform the things you eat into simple numbers. All you need to do is track them and increase or decrease your daily intake of them depending on whether you want to increase or decrease your weight. When I began to understand this concept, I wondered how it could be so simple and still work, and how the fitness industry could be lying to all of us with its complicated, expensive solutions for staying slim and fit. Then I remembered: *Oh yeah, because they want our money!*

IT'S NOT THE BANANAS. IT'S NOT THE TUNA.

It was such a relief to find so many talented people on social media providing so much value and giving back a ton of honest information solely for the purpose of helping others. It was such a relief after my experience in the gym for so many years. It also reinforced to me that natural bodybuilders have a much more sustainable system for the average person than a professional who uses performance-enhancing drugs.

From constantly following these natural bodybuilders, I was able to understand their day-to-day lives and realize that you can't just take a magic pill, or take some injection, to stay in shape. You've got to put effort into it. So many of us want to believe that the successful people of the world are taking shortcuts we'll never have access to. We'll say, "That person knows something I don't know," or "He's drinking some special drink that I can't afford."

Don't have that fucking attitude. There's a book I recommend by renowned psychologist Carol Dweck entitled Mindset: The New Psychology of Success. In it, she writes that people too often go through life with a fixed mindset. They don't open their world to new possibilities, can never see themselves in a new light, and avoid challenges and the possibility of failure.

To succeed, though, you need a growth mindset. You should embrace new challenges, and with hard work and time, you can reach new levels of higher achievement. You just have to believe that you can get there through persistence. I agree with Dweck that building blocks to your success are out there. They're free, and they're right in front of your eyes. Yes, becoming slimmer, fitter, and healthier requires commitment, hard work, and discipline. But the rewards are longer lasting and a million times greater than anything you can shoot into your butt with a syringe made for a bull. As the great Marcus Aurelius once said, "The impediment to action advances action. What stands in the way becomes the way."

I've put all of the building blocks together in this book. I have expanded on the work of the many sources mentioned here, along with that of many others, to form Lean Life. The material collected is the result of my own fitness failures and successes.

With it, you'll be able to gain maximum fitness and health in the most time-efficient way possible. It will save you from the aggression, mania, weepiness, and other side effects of magic pill solutions. It will stop falling-outs with friends and violent addictions that will ruin your life. Or was that just me?

Regardless, in the coming chapters, I'll be placing a buffet table full of information in front of you. On the first serving dish is the concept of tracking your macros. On the second is Intermittent Fasting. On the third is Reverse Pyramid training. How you dig into them—together or in separate pieces, large servings or small—is up to you.

If you try all three portions of the Lean Life system together, you'll most likely get amazing results. You might even see the 50 percent improvement in weight strength, 50 percent reduction in body fat, and 100 percent improvement in health and happiness that I got. Maybe you'll do even better. Try two of them together, and you'll still get great results. Try one of them, and your results will still be extremely positive. Just remember, you receive benefits in proportion to what you put into the program. It's not the bananas and tuna; it's you.

Takeaways

- Macronutrients are types of food needed in large amounts in your diet. They are fats, proteins, and carbohydrates.
- Natural bodybuilding is the concept of lifting weights to increase strength and muscle definition without the use of performance-enhancing drugs.
- It's important to listen to natural athletes for practical advice as well as setting realistic goals, as opposed to listening to those who are using special substances to give them amazing results.

Recommended Reading

- *Mindset: The New Psychology of Success* by Carol Dweck

2

Saved from the Stinking Chicken

*There's no such thing as failure—
just giving up too soon.*

–Dr. Jonas Salk

PICTURE, FOR A SECOND, your typical chubby, out-of-shape teenaged social outcast, and you're basically imagining me fourteen years ago. I lived in Temple, Texas, population fifty-five thousand, an hour north of Austin where the big weekend hobby for teenagers consisted of drinking beer and smoking weed. Being someone who wanted to fit in, I joined the crowd. But since I wasn't very stealthy, my parents kept busting me. Every time I was caught partying, they'd yell at me and take away the keys to my car, a used 1997 Toyota Corolla. The only place they'd let me go when I was grounded was to the gym—because it involved exercise, and they figured I wouldn't be socializing with anyone there.

The gym closest to me was the local recreation center, where the only people who worked out were senior citizens and dudes who didn't seem very interested in finding jobs. I'd go there because it was close by and allowed me to get out of the house.

At that point in time, I followed the normal "bro" routine of blasting one body part a day—chest, back, arms, shoulders, legs—then I'd hit the sauna and go home. Rinse and repeat.

Before long, I started enjoying the routine and being in better shape. I even got to know some of the old folks and creepy unemployed guys working out there. I went to the gym four or five days a week, and as part of every workout, I ran two miles on the treadmill. Afterward, I'd sit on a chair for ten minutes to lower my heart rate and then lift weights. Even after my parents lifted my social restrictions, I kept going.

Over the course of the next several months, the weight started falling off of me, despite my ignorance with weights and fitness. I wanted to get even leaner, so I changed my nutrition habits and stopped eating carbohydrates altogether. That's right, no bread or rice or anything. For snacks, I'd put turkey slices and cucumbers into a Tupperware container and carry it in my backpack with an apple and a protein shake.

The next thing I knew, I looked in the mirror and saw a really skinny five-foot-six, 120-pound kid with a 28-inch waist. I'd lost more than 20 pounds, and I liked what I had become. So did girls. They started talking to me, and I started to go out and have more fun. I got my first girlfriend, and girls wanted to have sex with me. I was sixteen years old and thought, "This is amazing!"

What I didn't realize at the time was that I was doing too much cardio and not eating enough carbs. My diet wasn't sustainable. Think about eliminating carbs for a second. Do you really expect a person to go carb-free for the rest of his or her life? The real reason cutting carbs works is because you're simply eating fewer calories when you do it. In the end, it's all about calorie intake. Decreasing calories = weight loss. If you start eating the carbs again, you're going to gain that weight again.

More important to weight control is portion control. When you cut carbs, it depletes glycogen. So much of the weight you lose is simply water weight anyway. When you reintroduce carbs, you gain that weight back.

HOW MOST PEOPLE THINK LOW CARB DIETS WORK

HOW LOW CARB DIETS ACTUALLY WORK

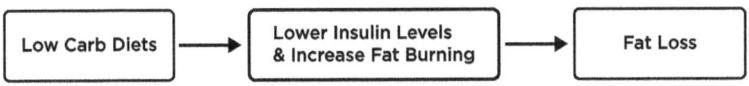

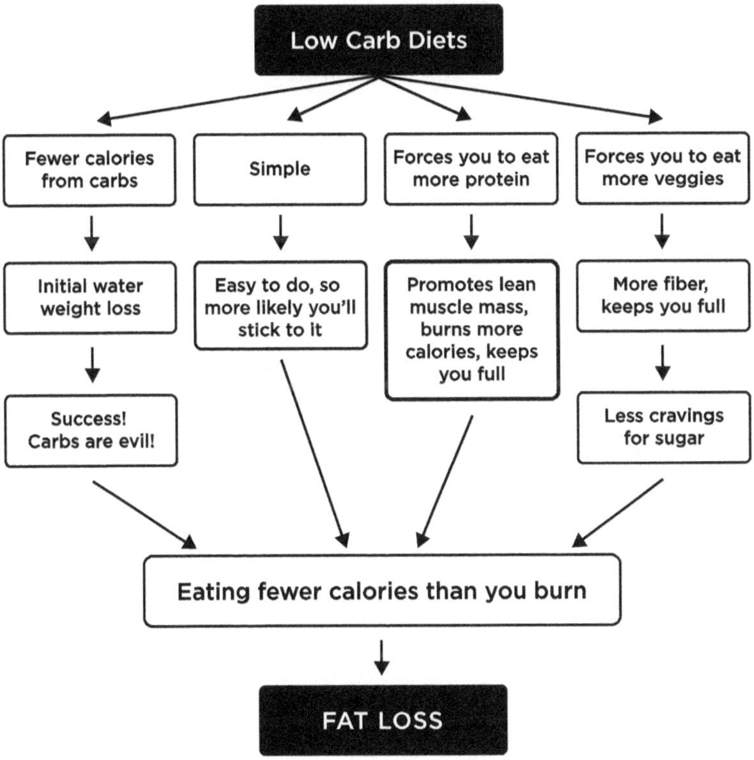

The weight-loss results I had achieved at that time came mostly from the carb cutting, and running. So I kept at the cardio, doing the two miles a day. The treadmill had this little display of a quarter-mile track that lit up as you went along until you made your way fully around it. I always had it in my mind to do this eight times. I have no idea why two miles. It just seemed like a good distance.

The running had another positive effect: it enticed me to quit smoking so I could breathe better for the workouts. The improvement was almost instant, as my heart and lungs quickly started feeling much stronger and I could run faster. I quit smoking cigarettes completely and only smoked weed because it didn't seem as bad, and I didn't do it as much.

The problem with going to a crappy gym where mostly only creepy people work out is that they're the only ones at your disposal to give you exercise tips. One time, an old guy came up to me and said, "Every time you come into the gym, do a 'push' exercise and then a 'pull' one. Then, by the time you're my age, you'll be twice my size!"

I was an impressionable kid and willing to do anything that a mentor-figure told me to try. So I thought, "OK! Yes! Push weights, pull weights." But after trying it a few times, I realized he left out a lot of other pieces of the puzzle. What specific exercises to do? How many reps? What weight to use? Which muscles? Again, I was given a piece of a puzzle, but not a straightforward plan on what to do in a gym. What shitty advice to give a sixteen-year-old without offering the full picture!

Between the bad advice and my own teenage ignorance, I was making a lot of mistakes with my nutrition and fitness. There was no such thing as social media to help me out. There was no large, unified community of people connected by hashtags who were staying fit and sharing their knowledge and information for free in the way that they do today. The Internet was only good for looking at porn and plagiarizing papers for history class at that time. So instead, I got all of my knowledge from *Men's Health* articles. I'd pull out the posters of the really chiseled models jumping on a box, or doing something else I didn't want to do, and hang them up. Then I never followed the exercises, or I tried them only briefly. The one part of my routine I did do correctly was drink a lot of water. I carried around a bottle that I filled all the time.

The single biggest mistake I made as a teenager was not understanding that the process of becoming sounder in mind and body is a discipline. Life itself is a discipline. That's why you find all of those inspirational posters with the word "discipline" on them. They're clichés because they're true. "Discipline is just choosing between what you want now and what you want most," is a big one. And, "Suffer the pain of discipline, or suffer the pain of regret." And, my favorite, "Discipline is the bridge between goals and accomplishments."

I wanted discipline, but the second girls started wanting to date me when I lost weight, it stopped because the destination had become more important than the journey. The destination was everything I saw on the cover of *Men's Health*: Six-pack abs now. Have more sex. Put more money in your pocket. Once I got some of those things, I stopped being committed to the sources of my success.

That's the difference with me today. All of that stuff from the *Men's Health* cover is great, but it's not why I created and follow Lean Life, and it's not what motivates me. Getting in better shape and going to the gym are emotional decisions you make. You have to be honest with yourself to understand what's motivating you, what the underlying change is that you want to make for your body. Whether it's the sixteen-year-old me who wants a better body, which is why most people are drawn to the gym, or the mature version of me who wants to simply stay healthy and live a life of balance and moderation. Now the journey is everything for me, and maintaining self-discipline is the ultimate success. Without discipline you can't overcome your struggles, or maintain a healthy self.

The turning point, as I've mentioned, came in Egypt. But before that happened, I made plenty of mistakes. One of them was the chicken-and-rice diet. My life was pretty hectic at the time. It was early in my med school years, before my steroid debacle.

During the day, I took my regular course load, and at night, as part of the med school system in Egypt, I took evening tutoring classes taught by professors. Each one was two hours long, and two of them were scheduled back-to-back twice a week, Monday through Thursday. For example, on a typical Monday and Wednesday, I might have anatomy from 7:00 p.m. to 9:00 p.m. and then physiology from 9:00 p.m. to 11:00 p.m. Then on Tuesday and Thursday, I'd have biochemistry and histology during those same time blocks. On top of all that, I started doing stand-up comedy on the side. Sleep was an idea, but not much of a reality for me. I was completely overextended and stopped taking care of myself.

I even started smoking again. Cigarettes are everywhere in Egypt. Even a lot of my professors were smokers, which was ironic. But in the Middle East, it's a deeply rooted cultural thing. I also ate total junk, like whatever fried stuff was sold from carts on the street. And when I say junk, I actually mean it. In Egypt, it's common to get gastroenteritis—better known as vomiting or the shits—from street food. I've even known classmates who have gotten hepatitis from it.

I found that it was hard to exercise self-control in a society that focused so much on eating. There was so much great food around me all of the time—on the streets and in restaurants and cafes. You only have so much willpower when you're hungry in that type of environment and you don't have a structured and disciplined eating plan. It's harder to make good choices when there's so much convenience.

In the United States, you see similar dangers with fast food. You've got all of these delicious, deep-fried goodies available to you at a drive-through window whenever you need it. Chain restaurants aren't concerned with whether you lose weight. They're trying to sell a product, and it's food. They're going to make it highly palatable, and super cheap, whether you have self-control or not.

The irony was that healthy food was inexpensive over there, as well. Tomatoes cost nothing—like ten cents a pound. Fruits like figs and pomegranates are sold cheaply, too. Produce is plentiful because Egyptians are farmers. They're on the Nile and the culture there was born on farming. They eat a lot of fava beans, which aren't nearly as popular in the rest of the world but are easy to grow in that region. Yet fast food is still proliferating in the Middle East right now.

One of my favorite Egyptian meals is called Ful Medames, which combines olive oil, garlic, cumin, lemon, and fava beans. You slow cook it, dip pita bread in it, and eat it with your hands. It's low cost and easy. I could have made it all the time if I wanted. Red meat is expensive, so Egyptians stick mostly to vegetables, legumes, and fish.

Because of the high-pressure, bad-eating, up-all-night, no-exercising lifestyle of graduate students in general in Egypt, taking care of themselves takes a back seat. I lived this experience firsthand. It becomes very easy to get out of shape. But then again, you'll find that anywhere. Compared to most of my peers, I was fit—but not by my standards. Balancing everything was hard, and I squeezed in workouts when I could, carrying my gym stuff in a bag wherever I went.

After a while, I knew I had to change my eating habits to stay trim, and I had to get off the street food. I tried to follow a healthy diet, but went about it the wrong way by following the ways of "bro" science. I made the tragic mistake of going on a chicken-and-rice diet. Only chicken and rice and broccoli. Nothing else. Brilliant, right? Dr. Juice told me about it, for some reason, before he became my drug dealer, and I listened. Hey, he was a medical professional—a dentist, right? Besides, it sounded better than tuna and bananas.

For my meals, I'd get a kilogram (That's 2.2 pounds) of chicken breast, cut it up, boil it, and then make a pot of rice to go with it. It sucked. Yet I found myself putting the chicken and rice in a Tupperware container and carrying it with me because I didn't think I could eat anything else.

I believed in the myth of eating six meals a day to boost my metabolism. I thought that smaller, more frequent eating sessions would force the body to burn more calories simply to digest the food I was eating. This was a skewed interpretation of science. I now know that the thermogenic effect of food, or TEF, dictates that the amount of calories it takes to digest food is directly proportional to the amount of food you eat, not the frequency of meals.

I remember that often before performing in a stand-up show, I'd sit on a bench in a far, hidden corner backstage or in the alley behind the club, shoveling chicken and rice into my mouth as

SAVED FROM THE STINKING CHICKEN

I waited to go on. I was too embarrassed to let anyone see how much of a "bro" I was. Everything in my food container would be mush, but I'd stick a fork in it. If I lingered long enough, stray cats would come and sit next to me, begging for food. The thought that always went through my mind was, *This is my life. Sitting with stray cats and eating alone. Awesome.*

It's funny, because when I see house cats now, it reminds me of those chicken-and-rice moments. People here don't know how bad conditions can be in developing countries, for humans and animals to survive. I'll make fun of house cats and say, "You should see your brothers and sisters that are out there begging for anything they can get."

With people and cats, there's one way we're all the same, though, no matter the location: we'll eat whatever's easiest and most convenient. For cats, it's whatever is in a garbage can. For us, it's from the McDonald's or wherever. I was trying to pry myself from the convenience trap I had fallen into in Egypt, but approaching it the wrong way. Chicken and rice wasn't the answer, I eventually understood that—but not until after some suffering, though.

The solution eventually came to me during my research in my post-steroid funk: the hashtag IIFYM, and the concept of macronutrients. From my science and medical background, I knew what a macronutrient was. It's a $10,000 word for a substance that gives you the calories (or energy) your body needs to function. The "macro" part means that it makes up a majority of your diet.

There Are Three Basic Macros:

1. Protein
2. Carbohydrates
3. Fat

Fiber is sometimes considered the fourth macro, for good reason too; it helps keep you full, "regular," and ensures that you're eating your fruits and veggies. Just make sure and get a decent amount in your diet. The recommended daily amount for adults is twenty-five to thirty grams.

Protein and carbohydrates have four calories per gram. Fat has nine calories per gram. So in equation form (I hate math more than you, but relax, there's no calculus, just basic math)

4P + 4C + 9F = Total Calories

Let's see what this means in practice. Note the calories and macros on the following label:

Kellog's® Pop-Tarts® Frosted Strawberry

Nutrition Facts

Serving Size 1 Pastry (52g)

Amount per Serving

Calories 200   Calories from Fat 45

	% Daily Value*
Total Fat 5g	8%
Saturated Fat 1.5g	8%
Trans Fat 0g	
Polysaturated Fat 2g	
Monosaturated Fat 1g	
Cholesterol 0mg	0%
Sodium 170mg	7%
Total Carbohydrate 38g	13%
Dietary Fiber less than 1g	3%
Sugars 16g	
Protein 2g	

Vitamin A 10% · Vitamin C 0% · Calcium 0% · Iron 10%
Thiamin 10% · Riboflavin 0% · Niacin 0% · Vitamin Bc 10%

* Percent Daily Values are based on a 2,000 calorie diet. Your daily values may be higher or lower depending on your caloric needs.

	Calories	2,000	2,500
Total Fat	Less than	65g	80g
Saturated Fat	Less than	20g	25g
Cholesterol	Less than	300mg	300mg
Sodium	Less than	2,400mg	2,400mg
Dietary Fiber		25g	30g

The label shows 230 calories, 3 grams protein, 37 grams carbs, and 8 grams fat, so

(4 x 3) + (4 x 37) + (9 x 8) = calories,

12 + 148 + 72 = 232 calories.

As I wrote earlier, there are three basic macronutrients: carbohydrates, proteins, and fats. (I should point out that fiber and alcohol are also sometimes considered macronutrients, but to make things easy, we won't be referring to them here.) Carbohydrates are the main fuel that keeps the furnace burning in our bodies. Proteins build and preserve muscle mass, strengthen our immune systems and healing, and preserve muscle. Fats store energy and are important for the structural integrity of cells as well as absorbing vitamins. By contrast, micronutrients are the substances our bodies need in smaller amounts, such as vitamins and minerals.

IIFYM stands for "If it fits your macros." It was a regular hashtag used on posts by some of the people I had begun following on Instagram. They'd write something about the meal they just ate and include a code such as 12 F, 50 C, 25 P and then put #IIFYM next to it.

I thought, *What is this strange hieroglyphic language?* So I dug deeper and found out more. The basic philosophy behind it goes like this: It takes calorie counting to the next level by tracking each macronutrient. So you're calculating the grams of fat, carbs, and proteins at the end of each day. After you adjust your calories and macros according to your goals, your diet simply becomes a numbers game. If you want to lose weight, you'd simply lower your intake of carbs and fat.

IIFYM, or flexible dieting, is just that. It's a flexible approach that allows you to choose your diet, within reason. So it doesn't make any difference whether your macros come from

SAVED FROM THE STINKING CHICKEN

a deep-fried Twinkie or a kale-and-lentil smoothie. Or even a Pop-Tart (but more on this later). All that matters is that if you stay under your set macro and calorie limit for the day, you'll lose weight without a problem. Of course, you'll want to rely mostly on healthy, natural foods rather than processed foods.

In those IIFYM hieroglyphics I was reading on people's Instagram posts, I discovered the letter "f" stood for fat, "c" for carb, and "p" for protein. The numbers represented amounts consumed, and the key was to count every one of them throughout the day.

The reason natural, unprocessed, unfried foods help you lose weight isn't because they're "healthier" by nature—though they are. It's because they're not packed with as many macros or calories as a plate of nachos with Cheez Whiz on top, so you can eat more of them without blowing through your daily load of carbohydrates, fat, and protein at one time. They "fit" your daily macro allowance easier, and whole natural foods are more filled with micronutrients, which people classify as "healthier" choices. What's often not understood, though, is that you can still overeat "healthy" foods and gain weight, which can cause frustration.

When I learned the philosophy behind the people posting #IIFYM, a whole new world opened up to me. They were telling me, through pictures, go eat donuts, go eat a cheeseburger, but within reason. Eat whatever the fuck you want if you can fit it into your macro count. At times, you do need to be strict, of course, but not restrictive. Don't get me wrong, I'm not saying you can eat thirty donuts and a cheeseburger every day. I actually found out the hard way that this is the wrong way for you to start flexible dieting. Some people believe IIFYM encourages a complete junk food diet. It doesn't. The flexibility and fun lies in the 10 to 30 percent leeway in your diet that allows for the treats that with other diet plans you generally have to keep out of your mouth unless you're on a cheat day.

From that point, I began following the accounts of popular IIFYM gurus such as Kane Sumabat (@timbahwolffff on Instagram); Layne Norton (@biolayne), who's a professional powerlifter with a PhD in nutritional science; Jorge Rosado (@fitness_iq), a national physique competitor who was Mr. Florida 2013; and Mike Vacant @mikevacanti, as well as Brandon Carter. I learned a lot about the flexible dieting approach from them and scoured everything I could on the subject on Instagram, YouTube, websites, and online tutorials.

Instant messaging became my friend, as well. For answers to specific questions, I contacted a few people who were dedicated to IIFYM but didn't have huge, insanely popular online profiles. I figured they were more likely to answer back. One of the most responsive people was Tony TBone Somera, who has the Instagram handle @SuperSaiyanTbone. He posts tons of pictures of the things he eats, like big ice cream cones or chocolate-covered donuts with sprinkles, along with selfies of himself in a tank top showing how lean and cut he is. The two of us messaged back and forth a lot, and he was great at giving me guidance.

He and some of my other #IIFYM mentors told me that there are two important aids that help in successful macro tracking. The first is the app MyFitnessPal, which is endorsed by many dietitians and doctors and has over five million foods in its database. It can instantly spit out the nutritional information on whatever food you're eating, and track your calories throughout the day, week, month, and year. It even has a barcode scanner so you can pick up an item at the supermarket and immediately know its calories and macronutrients.

The other important tool is a food scale to measure exact serving sizes for the food you prepare yourself. I knew exactly where I could get one. My dad is a big stamp collector, and he kept postage scales that were super accurate for sending letters or packages. The next time I went home to the United States for a med school break, I grabbed one.

Finally I was ready to test the #IIFYM methods. My mentors set me straight on the basics—like creating my macro limits based on my weight and physical activities, and they offered plenty of tips and advice—all without charge, because they just wanted to pass along the knowledge to grow the community and improve people's lives. Teamwork makes the dream work, baby!

When I got back to Cairo, I became an obsessive macro counter. I'm the type of person who, if I'm going to do something, I'm going all in. One of the perks of being in the United States is that most anything with a barcode can be found in MyFitnessPal. Unfortunately, in Egypt, even the groceries with bar codes weren't updated. So I had to stick to mostly whole foods, I actually had to weigh most of what I was eating, which was time consuming at first, but fine. I measured everything from Basmati rice to bananas to chicken breasts—all the way down to the gram. Then I plugged everything into MyFitnessPal.

You'll find, as I did, that the first few weeks can be overwhelming, but as soon as you start getting into a system of repetition, and MyFitnessPal has already recorded most of your meals, it gets a lot easier. And after a while, you get very good at knowing the values of portion sizes without a scale. I've been counting macros for so long, now, I can tell how many grams a food is just by looking at it.

My transition to tracking my macros only tells half the story of how I changed my eating habits—for the better—in med school. The other is Intermittent Fasting, which also has a big following among most of those who follow #IIFYM or flexible dieting, including Kane Sumabat and Tony Somera. It's the practice of fasting for an extended period of the day, like sixteen hours and then eating all your food during the rest of the time.

The great aspect about fasting, similar to the flexible diet approach is that it doesn't restrict you from any foods. It's simply about timing when you eat. The only real way to lose weight is through prolonged calorie restriction, and fasting is a great tool that allows you do to that.

Fasting is purposely abstaining from calories. You'll discover that there's not a lot of research on the subject because most research on eating habits is funded by the food industry. They're certainly not going to delve into the benefits of skipping meals. Instead, literally billions of dollars are spent on ads and research to tell you to eat and not to fast. Fasting, however, takes away the needless sacrifice of dieting and shows incredible results for keeping you slim given you're staying within your calorie/macro count.

People wrongly think they'll lose muscle mass when they fast. Yet studies have shown that as long as they lift weight and get sufficient protein in their diets, their muscle mass is preserved. Fasting is great because it allows you to adhere more easily to calorie and macro restrictions since your window for eating during the day is smaller.

All effective diets may work simply because—at the end of the day—they restrict your overall calorie intake. But most are hard to follow for an extended period of time because they focus on cutting out certain foods or excessively adding others. My weight fluctuated over the years because I had tried so many of them.

Intermittent Fasting, however, allowed me to maintain a calorie deficit because I was able to eat the foods I liked and enjoy large meals. Meanwhile, I was decreasing weight, maintaining muscle mass, decreasing blood glucose and insulin levels, and increasing insulin sensitivity and production of growth hormones. Just as importantly, it was also enhancing lipolysis.

Important fasting-related terms to know:

Lipolysis: A $10,000 word for burning fat. During fasting, your muscles oxidize fatty acids for fuel, which is great because when most people want to lose weight, what they don't realize is that they really want to lose fat and maintain muscle mass. After fasting for up to twenty-four hours, there's an increase of lipolysis up to 50 percent.

Glucagon: A hormone that helps regulate blood sugar in the body. When you're in a fasted state, glucagon is high.

Epinephrine and norepinephrine: They are your fight or flight hormones, and they actually facilitate the release of glucose from energy stores when fasting, which sparks fat burning. They also keep you alert.

How does fat burning, or lipolysis, work while fasting? Allow me to put on my doctor's white coat for a moment: Let's say your liver is your body's gas tank. It holds your glycogen, which is the gas. Whenever you eat, you're filling the tank with glycogen. In general, it takes about twenty-four to forty-eight hours for that gas tank to reach "empty." After that point, with no sugar left to burn, your body starts burning fat instead. After glycogen is depleted, your body starts using fat energy.

You might hear people throw around terms such as "fat oxidation," which is just a $150,000 word to explain burning fat. Go back thousands of years and hunter-gatherers would hunt, fast for extended periods of time, kill an animal, eat, and then repeat the cycle. They didn't have snacks in their pockets or refrigerators to store their meals. They were forced to intermittent fast. The human body is built to handle—and even thrive—on it.

Now let's think about the car analogy again for a second. You've just gone to the gas station—or eaten a meal—and then you drive fifty miles. Are you rushing to fill up the tank again? No. The most efficient thing to do is wait till the tank empties first. The same goes for eating.

Potential Benefits of Fasting

Studies on lab animals show that fasting has all sorts of side benefits, among them are the following:

It potentially stimulates the growth of new nerve cells and increases brain hormone levels, which could delay the onset of Alzheimer's disease or reduce its severity.

It has anti-aging properties and could prolong life.

On the digestive side, your body will thank you too. Your gastrointestinal tract is huge. It consists of your stomach and intestines, and is where your body digests food, absorbs nutrients, and gets rid of waste. It extends about thirty feet long in the average human. Think of the amount of blood that needs to go to this area when you're digesting—just so you can use the toilet—and the hormones and enzymes that need to be secreted as part of the process.

That's why, when people are eating all day, they're farting and pooping constantly and want to take a nap, like a baby. In a fasted state, the gastrointestinal tract sends waves of electrical activity—every ninety minutes to two hours—through the system to cleanse it of undigested material. The fancy name for this process is migrating myoelectric complex. An unfancy thing for you to know about it is that it keeps your bowels regular. When I was doing my rounds during my intern year, there were only two things older men cared about: getting an erection and being able to poop. Intermittent Fasting takes care of number two on the list, so to speak.

So how do you set up your own fasting protocol? There are many different methods to Intermittent Fasting. Two of the more popular ones are Lean Gains and Warrior Diet methods. They promote daily fasting. You can pick from an eating window of ten, eight, six, or even four hours.

As an example, let's use the sixteen hours of fasting, eight hours of eating, or 16/8, protocol. Note the fasting period includes when you sleep, so the eight hours is not as bad as it appears. Let's say you last ate at 10:00 p.m. You're not going to be eating until 2 p.m. the next day, and your window will last for another eight hours. The important thing is that you abstain from calories completely during the fasting time. You can drink water, take multivitamins, and have coffee and diet drinks, but no calories.

After a few days, once your body becomes acclimated, you'll realize how easy Intermittent Fasting can be to maintain. Because I'm used to the routine, I can go longer than sixteen hours without eating if I want. Sometimes it feels nice to stretch the fasting into overtime. In my mind I'll be saying, *I'm burning fat now, I like this!* Then when I'm ready, I'm free to eat. If it's a workout day, I'll go to the gym before that, because I like to exercise in a fasting state.

When I eat, I eat just about anything as long as it fits my macros. I've got twenty-two hundred calories at my disposal, almost. It's like saving your paycheck; you're not spending your money on a bunch of stuff all day, so then you have this large amount to spend at once. You have more to work with.

On the surface, Intermittent Fasting may seem restrictive. But in practice, it's quite liberating. It's strict but not restrictive. I find it easier simply not to eat in the morning, instead of worrying about what snacks I can and can't have. When you're in the office and everyone is bringing in a ton of food, it's tough to measure all of the calories and macros. From a practical standpoint, it's simply easier to simply fast and not deal with any of it until you dig into the choices you've prepared and brought with you.

I remember first trying to fast in Egypt, and it immediately felt like the best thing I'd ever done. I felt a sense of liberation because I was able to ditch the chicken and rice and enjoy the food I prepared at home. When I think of all of the gimmicky diets I tried, I'm embarrassed now. It was done out of ignorance because I didn't understand that these diets worked simply because of the golden rule, which is calorie restriction.

IIFYM on social media can be misleading because you only see the 10 percent of a person's diet that consists of junk. But you don't see what's behind the curtain, which is the healthy whole food that comprises the other 90 percent. Which brings me to my Pop-Tarts story. It explains how and why I got into Intermittent Fasting in the first place.

The nutritional information on a single frosted strawberry Pop-Tart reads like this:

Kellog's® Pop-Tarts® *Frosted Strawberry*

Nutrition Facts

Serving Size 1 Pastry (52g)

Amount per Serving

Calories 200   Calories from Fat 45

	% Daily Value*
Total Fat 5g	8%
Saturated Fat 1.5g	8%
Trans Fat 0g	
Polysaturated Fat 2g	
Monosaturated Fat 1g	
Cholesterol 0mg	0%
Sodium 170mg	7%
Total Carbohydrate 38g	13%
Dietary Fiber less than 1g	3%
Sugars 16g	
Protein 2g	

Vitamin A 10% · Vitamin C 0% · Calcium 0% · Iron 10%
Thiamin 10% · Riboflavin 0% · Niacin 0% · Vitamin Bc 10%

* Percent Daily Values are based on a 2,000 calorie diet. Your daily values may be higher or lower depending on your caloric needs.

	Calories	2,000	2,500
Total Fat	Less than	65g	80g
Saturated Fat	Less than	20g	25g
Cholesterol	Less than	300mg	300mg
Sodium	Less than	2,400mg	2,400mg
Dietary Fiber		25g	30g

This is for one Pop-Tart, and there are two in a pack, which is what the average person will eat. Not exactly a health food is it?

I remember this one stand-up routine by Jerry Seinfeld. In it, he would talk about how he got Pop-Tarts when he was a kid and they were so magical. It was hilarious. But really, in my eyes, Pop-Tarts were invented for parents who are too lazy to cook a proper breakfast and would be happy to buy this cardboard square thing that comes in an aluminum wrapper instead and just throw it in a toaster for forty-five seconds. When it comes out, they're basically saying," Here you go, child. This is your breakfast."

As an adult, would you care about a Pop-Tart? Would you take one if someone offered it to you? You'd be confused and say, "This is so infantile and immature." Yet here was this community of grown-ups eating them, and working out at the gym and posting pictures on social media, and I was thinking, *Is this a joke?*

It was real, but at the same time they were saying, "Hey, look at us getting away with eating this absolute garbage. You must be confused about how we're doing this because what we're doing is science based."

Even to this day, you'll see some people posting Pop-Tart pictures, though not as many. But at the time, when I was in Egypt, the Instagram posts I saw definitely made me say, "Holy shit! What are they doing? They're eating Pop-Tarts, and they're in great shape! Tell me more!"

As I got more practice at tracking macros and Intermittent Fasting, I jumped on the Pop-Tart train. The problem was that I was in Egypt, which isn't exactly Kellogg's Breakfast Pastry Central. To get them, I needed to make a special trip to one specific supermarket—located nowhere near where I lived—that imported internationally branded foods from other countries including, thankfully, Pop-Tarts. They were expensive, too, like flaky frosted gold.

Pop-Tarts are cheap as hell here, right? Maybe two bucks for a box of six. But over there the same thing cost eight dollars! Still, I went out and bought them, because I was thinking, *I need these for #IIFYM!*

I remember posting my first Instagram video feed of me eating one smothered in Nutella. There I was, in a developing country, with the world's most expensive Pop-Tart in my hands! I shortly realized that eating nine hundred calories that are low in micronutrients is great for laughs, but not for getting you full. Now for me, nine hundred calories means two nutritious meals with a lean protein source, potatoes, and fibrous veggies.

Many people make the mistake with Intermittent Fasting of fitting in the most junk they can squeeze into their eating window. That's not the approach they should take, though, especially as a beginner. Seventy to 90 percent is still whole foods. But the flexible diet still gives you the creativity to eat those snacks that you would usually save for a cheat day.

I discovered that tracking my macros was like entering the Matrix. I'd swallowed the red pill and from that day forward, all fats, carbs, and proteins were just numbers. All of these 0s and 1s were falling down around me—numbers that meant nothing when you looked at them separately, but filling the whole fabric of the universe when taken together.

What comes to my mind sometimes is that T-shirt that shows a drawing of a pipe, and above it are the French words, "Ce n'est pas une pipe," which in English means, "This is not a pipe." The idea is that the drawing is just a representation of a pipe, not the real thing. With my rendition of flexible dieting, we could almost make a T-shirt that says, "Ce n'est pas une

Pop-Tart." Because the Pop-Tart is just a symbol, telling you that you can eat whatever you like as long as it fits your macros.

Forget, too, the lies of the corporate fitness industry. So many malicious marketers are out there to sell you some magical pill that will instantly make you fitter, stronger, thinner—but these products really aren't good for anything except taking your money. The malicious marketers use your lack of knowledge against you and take advantage of people who feel vulnerable about how they look and what kind of shape they're in, and who are willing to try anything.

It's like the Nigerian prince who wants to share his fortune with you if you'll just send him your bank account number. The scammers who write these e-mails make them blatantly fake so that they'll only lure people who—for whatever reason—can't see through the complete bullshit. You can read more about this in the book *Think Like a Freak*, from the authors of Freakonomics.

The malicious fitness marketers are the same way. All of us can get so down about our appearance, and our state of health and fitness, that we're willing to try almost any easy answer, and sometimes we can't see through the most obvious bullshit. I was that way as a medical student. I believed Dr. Juice's nonsense about chicken and rice for that very reason! The malicious marketers will say, "Buy our product, and you'll get instant six-pack abs, or make more money, or have more sex." They know it plays to our emotional weaknesses and desires, and sadly it works.

The good news is that in this day and age, the world of information is changing; it's getting harder and harder to sell these magical pills. Now there are crowd-sourced online reviews for everything—from gas station toilets to fitness supplements. It's harder to lie about a product and get away with it because reviewers are lurking everywhere, and they have thumbs and they have smartphones, and they're going to tell the truth.

The Internet, especially social media, is so full of free useful content, too, from people who want to share their success stories and aren't trying to make millions of dollars off of you. That's where the best resources are found. That's also how I came upon Intermittent Fasting and #IIFYM, and formed the building blocks and inspiration for Lean Life, including Reverse Pyramid weight training.

My philosophy and approach to weight training has changed over the years and will continue to evolve, I'm sure. Most weight-lifting programs are beneficial. The golden rule for building muscle is "progressive overload," which means increasing weight, or sets and reps, over time, which is time consuming, ultimately.

Muscle & Strength Nutrition Pyramid

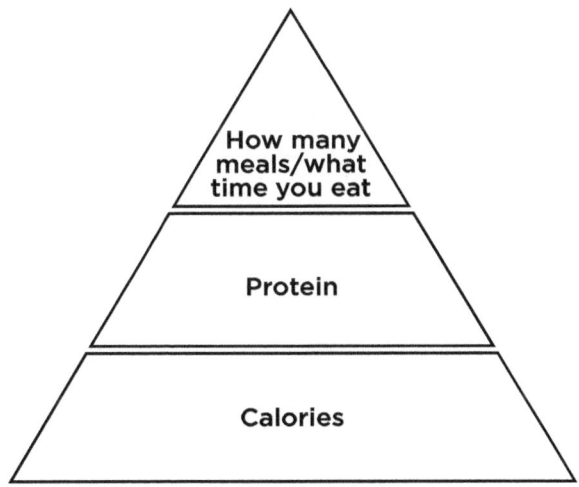

Muscle & Strength Training Pyramid

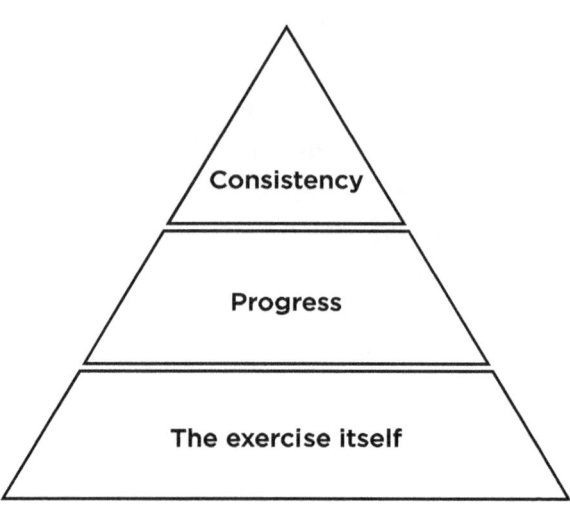

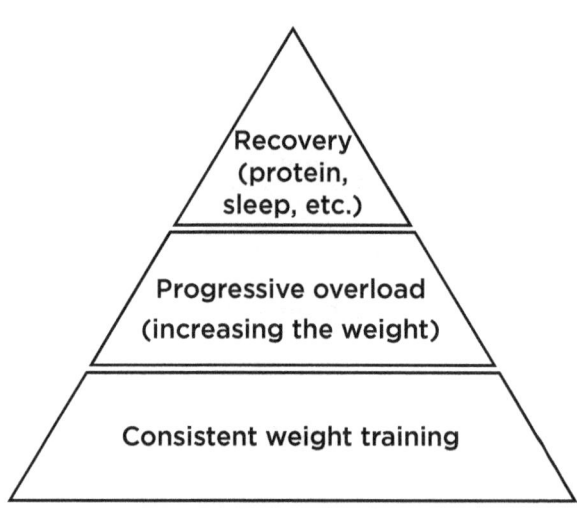

SAVED FROM THE STINKING CHICKEN

The whole concept behind the Reverse Pyramid training turns the conventional wisdom of lifting weights upside down. Most of us have been taught that a typical workout goes something like this: You do three to five sets of an exercise, with the weight going up—and the reps going down—for each set. Right? So someone who's bench-pressing might start with 12 reps at 150 pounds, then do the second set with 10 reps at 175 pounds, and the third at 8 reps and 200 pounds. Like I said, the weight up and the reps down. This method isn't wrong. However, upon discovering Reverse Pyramid training, I found that there is a more efficient way to stimulate muscle growth.

You want your muscles to exert the maximum amount of force possible when they're fresh, at the beginning of a workout, and then reduce the weight as they fatigue. So the first set has the fewest reps and heaviest weights. In each following set, you'll do progressively more reps with lower weights.

So let's say you start bench-pressing with seven reps at 200 pounds. Then you do the second set, decrease the weight 10 percent (to 180 pounds) and do one extra rep (seven reps). With Reverse Pyramid training, we're focusing on intensity or very heavy weight, basically. This kind of maximum stress on the muscle really helps you focus on strength and is one of the most efficient training regimes.

When people go to the gym and follow the traditional weight-training methods, by doing something like twelve, fifteen, or even twenty reps, they're not being as efficient and not taking advantage of the fact that they're in a place called a "weight" room. The higher the number of reps, the more the workout becomes aerobic (endurance and low intensity) instead of anaerobic (power driven and high intensity). You want to put a heavy stress load on the muscle—more than it has ever done before—to stimulate muscle fiber and promote maximum growth.

Don't get me wrong, if you follow any traditional-style, weight-training split, you can still get great results when sticking to a plan. But when you go through the motions with a traditional-style, weight-training session, unless you challenge yourself, you'll eventually hit a plateau because your muscles aren't being challenged enough if you don't eventually start using heavier weight. Reverse Pyramid taps into muscle power. It's much more efficient, too—getting you in and out of the gym faster but giving you better results.

The first time I tried the Reverse Pyramid approach, on the bench press, I couldn't believe how hard it was, because I'd never done anything like it. But the hurdle for me and most other beginners is mostly mental. I said to myself, "OK, this is a very heavy weight, but I have to make this go up and down six times, and I'm going to do it." Afterward, I had this immediate sense of confidence, because confidence always follows competence.

I enjoyed it so much. From that point, I was hooked, and I completely revised my workout routine and was able to stick to Reverse Pyramid training and make it a staple, along with counting macros and Intermittent Fasting. The foundation for Lean Life was already in place, though I didn't quite realize it yet. What I did realize was the immediate transformation my mind and body underwent.

Within the first four or five weeks of my early Lean Life experience, I was at least 50 percent stronger than I'd ever been, 50 percent leaner, and 100 percent happier and in a better place emotionally. I was able to spend less time in the gym, less time obsessing over what I ate, and more time on living my life and concentrating harder on medical school. I wasn't sitting in a

SAVED FROM THE STINKING CHICKEN

back alley behind a nightclub after performing a comedy routine and eating chicken and rice from a Tupperware container with stray cats by my side anymore. I was actually being social. This was three years ago, and the key from that point onward was understanding the roots of my transformation and maintaining self-discipline until Lean Life became a habit—a way of life.

As months passed, and my new routine became more of a way of life, I found I could get more lax in my approach. I could eyeball the measurements of some foods and stop carrying a scale around with me. Fasting became a lot easier. I customized my weight-lifting routines to fit my needs. Then I focused more clearly on my personal fitness and strength goals. Though I wanted to be strong and in great shape, my priority was to keep lean—not crazy lean, but enough so that I could take my shirt off at any time and still look good. I adjusted my approach to each of the three Lean Life pillars to achieve it. And it's a plan I stick with to this day.

Lean Life isn't a proprietary trade secret. Anyone can find and put together the same information that I did. But I'm sparing you, the reader, those years of Internet research I did; the countless hours I spent in med school classrooms learning the science behind the human body; and the fourteen-year trial-and-error learning process I went through, beginning when I was a chubby, socially maladjusted teenager lifting weights at the local recreation center in Temple, Texas.

I also hope to spare you from wasting your hard-earned money on bullshit supplements or other nonsensical garbage being thrown at you by the fitness industry. You have the power to choose what food you want to eat—you just need to do it at a more specific time and with a little bit of organization. You can be strict but not restrictive. As far as weight lifting goes, you don't need to waste an eternity at a commercial gym listening to a know-nothing trainer who's just there so he can stare at women's butts all day. You have the freedom to live your life.

In turn, you'll have a better sense of well-being. You'll be more confident in yourself—both in your appearance and your physical abilities. The Lean Life system is a strategic, science-based, logical approach that lets you focus on—and embrace—the moment and not worry so much on the end state. You'll start to enjoy the ride on the journey, which quickly becomes more important than the destination.

You won't be alone, either. There are millions of people who are using the three pillars of Lean Life in some capacity. There are a lot of community Facebook groups, where people are constantly checking in and holding each other accountable and sharing their progress with IIFYM, Intermittent Fasting, and weight training.

As you gain confidence, you can own your routines and regimens, and change them any way you like. They're not etched in stone. Lean Life is not a solution that only works a certain way. You're a highly capable person, and hundreds of millions of years of evolution has brought you to this beautiful moment. Nobody's telling you what to do. This book just helps give you small tools to help you build your own kingdom.

Don't feel the need to act on all three pillars of Lean Life either. Pick just two, or one. If you simply want to lose weight, you don't even need to set foot in a gym. Just follow the Intermittent Fasting and IIFYM approaches outlined in the later chapters here. Everybody's goals are very different. Some people really get bitten by the iron-pumping bug and do weight training for strength. Everybody's experience levels are different, and they will really dictate what the best weight-training program is for your tastes and needs. Embrace that you're shattering the conventions of the commercial fitness industry.

When I initially transitioned to Lean Life, the juicehead trainers at my gym in Egypt laughed at me. They saw me doing Reverse Pyramid training, and as I'd be walking out the door after thirty minutes they'd say, "What are you doing? You're not even working out."

I'd tell them I learned the workout online from a highly qualified personal trainer. Their answer: "You should stop reading stuff on the Internet!"

Seriously. That was their response. Stop reading. I thought, *Where am I living right now that people are telling me to stop reading?*

The people who saw me Intermittent Fasting in Cairo gave the same response. "You're crazy; you're stupid. You don't know what you're doing. It's the chicken and the rice! That's what works! It's the tuna and bananas! You have to eat them six times a day or your muscles will disappear!" For them, it's the same bullshit over and over again.

But a year into my Lean Life transition, they made no changes in their physiques; they weren't making progress in the weight they were lifting. They were stagnant. By comparison, I was leaner and stronger than I had ever been in my life. When people noticed my physical changes in the locker room, their imaginations got going. They were wondering if I was visiting Dr. Juice again. They couldn't believe that I could get such progress through natural sources.

"I'm not taking steroids," I'd say. "I'm doing the shit I told you about: Intermittent Fasting, tracking my macros, and Reverse Pyramid training." They refused to believe me. People always want to convince themselves that there's a secret answer out there that they don't know and can't ever get access to, and that's why they're not making progress.

Today, the aspect of Lean Life I've relied most upon is the fasting. I no longer micromanage my diet. I simply make sure I get a good amount of protein in, around one gram per pound of body weight, and then I eyeball the rest with carbs and fats. The gym is easy for me because I love working out—especially now that my sessions are shorter and more concentrated. It's a productive way for me to release stress.

My hope is that once you've taken the information in this book that fits your needs and lifestyle, you'll pass on your knowledge to others. In that way, you'll learn, you'll do, and then you'll teach. We're a community after all, and the more people we can save from the misery of chicken and rice, the better. I'm a minimalist. I want to get the best results in the least amount of time invested, and Lean Life is the way to do it.

Takeaways
- Macronutrients, or macros, are the required substances in food in order for humans to stay healthy. They are protein, carbohydrates, and fats. By tracking and controlling your macro intake, you can better control weight gain or loss.
- Intermittent Fasting is the act of refraining from the intake of calories for a set period of time each day or week in order to promote fat burning and weight loss.
- Reverse Pyramid weight training is a time-efficient weight-training protocol that involves putting the heaviest sets in a workout first to maximize intensity and strength.

3

Eat What You Want— Even Pop-Tarts

The more you eat, the less flavor;
the less you eat, the more flavor.
—Chinese Proverb

RICE AND CHICKEN! No, tuna and bananas! No, salmon and quinoa! No, Paleo! No, grapefruit only! I'm not going to tell you to stick to some fad diet. If I did, I'd be no better than those juicehead trainers in Cairo who made my life so miserable, or any other fitness guru who proclaims war on one specific macronutrient.

Fad diets work to a certain extent because the principle behind most of them is simply to restrict calories in order to reduce body fat. Any time you suddenly start eating less of a single macronutrient, you're going to be taking in fewer calories. The beauty of tracking macros isn't that it's a diet, per se. Instead, you're simply monitoring better what you're eating. It gives you freedom, within reason.

There's a misconception that the solution to looking fit and trim lies almost solely in working out at the gym. But that's actually only 20 percent of the equation. The other 80 percent is what you're putting into your mouth, your nutrition. Some people will go to the gym, work out really hard, and then drive to the Wendy's drive-through and order ten Baconators. Afterward they'll say, "Why am I not losing weight?" My answer: you can't out train a bad diet. Your emphasis should be on nutrition first. Nutrition is more important than an elliptical machine or Jazzercise. An hour of running or working out on an elliptical may only burn 300 or 400 calories, but your average combo meal exceeds 1,300 calories. You don't have enough time in the day to burn off this amount. Exercise is a secondary intervention to weight loss. The primary intervention is eating at a caloric deficit.

My best analogy for the 80-20, nutrition-to-workout ratio involves a bike and my favorite uncle. It goes like this: My favorite uncle visited my family from Egypt every year. He was chubby and funny, and just fun to be around. He'd always keep a stash of Pringles and Pepsi in the trunk of his car, and he would share some with me sometimes when he drove me places.

When I was around six years old, I had a lot of difficulty learning how to ride a bike. I was desperately trying to get rid of the training wheels, but couldn't seem to make the leap. But I was embarrassed because it just was not cool in the neighborhood to still have training wheels.

My uncle decided he would teach me how to ride a bike, so he took me to this really steep hill near my house. To me, it seemed like the Mount Everest of Temple, Texas. We walked all the way to the top, and my uncle told me to get on my bike. Then he crouched down and took the training wheels off.

"Those are for wimps," he told me as eh tossed them to the side. "Now, I tell you what you are going to do. You are going to try to stay on the bike."

The next thing I knew, he was pushing me down the hill. It scared the shit out of me, but I rode all the way to the bottom. I couldn't stop when I got there, so I crashed and skinned my knees. But by throwing me into the fire, he forced me to master the balance portion of riding.

My uncle knew that balance was 80 percent of learning to ride. The other 20 percent was pedaling. If he had taken me somewhere flat, like in a park, I would have had to master both elements at the same time. The learning curve would have been a lot longer. As soon as I got the hang of balance that day, though, pedaling was easy. He took me to the top of the hill a few more times, and pretty soon I was able to keep riding after the road plateaued at the bottom of the hill.

So how does this apply to getting leaner? As I wrote at the start of this chapter, there are two parts of the equation—nutrition and working out. Nutrition is the balance, the 80 percent. Working out is the pedaling, or the 20 percent. You'll need both, of course, so that your journey to fitness will be enjoyable like a bike ride.

Some people have more experience pedaling than others and that's great. But let's first focus on the most important thing, the balance, since that's the 80 percent. Let's kick the training wheels off those cookie-cutter diet plans that tell you to eat boiled chicken and broccoli and no carbs. That's garbage. Forget about them. You're an adult. It's time to push you down that fucking hill.

I know what you're asking: "Well, what can I eat?" On non-training days, I always stick to lower-carb options and eat more vegetables. On training days, I have more leeway to eat more carbs. No matter the day, I always include high protein. I'm not bound by this regimen, though. Eating great (and even sometimes terrible) food is one of the joys of life. You should embrace the opportunity, not deprive yourself of it—but in a smart way.

For me, I love street foods because of the variety of tastes and the cultural experience. The food in America is the best in the world. I even sometimes think the Thai or Middle Eastern cuisine we get here can be better than in the countries of origin themselves. Food is so excellent in the United States that it's the reason why so many people from other countries gain a lot of weight when they move here.

Austin is one of the country's culinary hotspots, and I take full advantage—tasting the world one forkful at a time. My favorite meal right now is jerk chicken sold from a Jamaican food truck near me. I also like just being able to grab a taco or a burger on the fly. When I'm cooking on my own, which is most of the time, I might make some salmon and quinoa or rice—something healthy and light. In my backpack I'll carry some high-protein bars.

On the days I do work out, I'll have more leeway in my diet and take in extra calories, not to make up for the energy I burn but simply because I'm weight training those days.

On the days I don't work out, I try to keep right at my calorie limit, maybe even a little bit below. That's really it. I don't micromanage anything. I've weaned myself off of obsessively tracking my macros. Unless you're one of those people who works out on stage or models their physique, it's a bit too much for you to count all of your calories in the long term. It's a short-term tool to get you to your ideal physique and to teach you how to portion control.

I'm a really big fan of whey protein powder. It's one of the most convenient, inexpensive, and high-quality protein sources out there. And it's a great way for me to ensure that I'm getting my daily allotted protein. Life is busy, and we have so many responsibilities—work, family, friends, social gatherings—that sometimes we don't have enough time to sit down and have a large enough meal to get all of our needed protein in.

Whey powders are another option to supplement your diet with protein. I order mine on Amazon for the cheapest price possible and they come in all sorts of crazy flavors, like birthday cake and snickerdoodle. I like to mix them with some Greek yogurt to make a kind of fat-free, low-carb pudding. Other great sources of protein are egg whites, cottage cheese, and lean meats like poultry (chicken or turkey breast), fish (salmon, tilapia), and lean beef cuts.

I'm not someone who tells you that you should only eat what falls from a plant or something. Instead, I consider myself a multivore—my own made-up name for people who eat whatever the hell they want. Even Pop-Tarts.

How can you be a multivore, too, and still stay lean? By tracking your macros. A "macronutrient," as I've mentioned, is a $10,000 word for the substances that give you the energy your body needs to function. There are three basic ones: carbohydrates, proteins, and fat. (Fiber is sometimes considered the fourth macronutrient, just make sure you get a good amount of it in your diet, fifteen grams per one thousand calories is a good rule of thumb.)

Carbohydrates fuel our bodies. They come in all forms, from complex, such as bread, rice, and pasta, to simple, such as table sugar or candy. There are four calories in one gram of carbohydrates.

No matter what, the carbs we eat are ultimately converted into glucose, which powers the muscles, brain, nervous system, tissues, and organs. When there's excess glucose in the body, it's stored as fat. And that's what we don't want.

Proteins are composed of amino acids, which are the building blocks for muscle, and also maintain your muscle mass and promote muscle protein synthesis. Poultry and fish are great sources of protein, as are egg whites and whey proteins. Vegetarians can find proteins in soy and beans, and they can also supplement their diets with protein supplements. There are four calories in one gram of protein.

Fat serves two important roles. First, fat absorbs vitamins essential for our nutrition and then sends them throughout our bodies. Second, it forms the padding that protects our organs and tissues and serves as the body's insulation. Additionally, fat provides fuel when the body runs out of available carbohydrates. Excessive saturated fats from fried foods, dairy, and meats can contribute to high cholesterol, which may lead to heart disease. Unsaturated fats are healthier and come from vegetable oils, nuts, and fish. There are nine calories in one gram of fat.

Before you can start down the #IIFYM path, you first need to know what your maintenance calories are.

Your recommended calorie intake—or basal metabolic rate (BMR)—is the golden key to figuring out how to unlock your macros. There are lots of BMR calculators on the Internet that can give you a decent estimate almost instantly.

Calories are the total units of energy that go into your body.

In order to give an example of typical maintenance calories, let's take an average Joe American who weighs 200 pounds and has a typical nine-to-five job at an office. To calculate his maintenance calories, we'll multiply his body weight times 13.5. That rounds to 2,700 calories. Those are Joe's maintenance calories. If he was to eat that amount of calories, he'd most likely stay the same weight. If Joe wants to lose weight, he'd eat less, if he wants to gain weight, he'd eat more. Obviously, Joe wants to lose weight. In order to lose weight, you need to be at a caloric deficit. Just a rule of thumb, one pound of fat = 3,500 calories.

EAT WHAT YOU WANT—EVEN POP-TARTS

So to lose one pound a week, you need to eat 3,500 calories less a week, or 500 calories less a day (3,500/7 days).

For Joe to lose one pound of fat a week, instead of 2,700 calories a day, he'd aim for 2,500 calories. From there, we'll calculate Joe's macronutrient composition for his diet. There are a lot of different ratios people use when dividing between proteins, fats, and carbohydrates. However, the most important thing is to start off by ensuring you get a good amount of protein. As we mentioned, we want Joe to get one gram of protein per pound of lean body weight (or goal bodyweight) so considering Joe has twenty pounds to lose and his idea body weight is 180, 180 grams of protein is how much Joe would aim for.

So if average Joe gets those 180 grams of protein a day, and we know one gram of protein has 4 calories in it, so 180 times 4 is 720. That means around 720 calories in Joe's daily diet should come from protein.

Now we can calculate how many grams of fat and carbs Joe would consume. Take 2,200 and subtract 720 and that gives us the remaining 1,480 calories he can divvy up between carbs and fat. For the sake of keeping things simple, average Joe just has to focus on those two concrete numbers: his total daily calories of 2,200 and approximately 180 grams of protein, if he wants to lose one pound of fat a week.

Let's say Joe wants to lose two pounds a week. Well, he'd aim for 1,800 calories daily and protein would stay the same at 180 grams a day.

Pretty simple, right? The key is being consistent and sticking with the numbers long enough.

Now you're probably asking why we didn't calculate the grams of fat and carbs for Joe. Well, the ratio of carbs and fat really isn't as important as his total calories and protein. If you just focus on those two numbers, you'll make things easier and also will allow for more flexibility around how many grams of carbs and fat you consume.

Here's a little cheat sheet for you, if you have fifty plus pounds of fat to lose and want to lose it as fast as reasonably possible (without cutting off a limb) use this nifty equation for superfast fat loss:

The Superfast Fat Loss Equation
You goal bodyweight in pounds x 10 = your daily calories

Your goal body weight in pounds x 1 = your daily grams of protein

Lean Life is based around flexibility: as long as your protein and calories are in check, you can get away with manipulating your carbs and fat to match your goals and preferences.

I emphasize maintaining protein because it's so essential for maintaining and building muscle and also keeps you full. I want you to keep it constant.

EAT WHAT YOU WANT—EVEN POP-TARTS

Breakfast	Calories kcal	Carbs g	Fat g	Protein g
Friendly Farms - Greek Yogurt - Plain, 2 cup (227 g)	260	18	1	46
Dymatize - Elite 100% Whey Protein Cookies & Cream, 69.8 g	260	6	3	50
Taylor Organic - Baby Spinach, 15 oz. (2o.)	100	15	0	10
Eggs - Whole Egg (1 white + 1 yellow), 4 egg	280	4	20	24
The Bakery - Soft Chocolate Chip Cookies, 2 cookie(s)	240	34	10	2
Milk - Reduced fat, 2% milkfat, 1 cup	122	11	5	8
Chicken - Breast, meat only, cooked, roasted, 100g	165	0	4	31
Bananas - Raw, 86g	77	20	0	1
Millville - Bran Flakes (Correct), 43.5g	165	36	1	5
Mahatma - Thai Jasmine Rice, 324g (cooked)	531	120	0	10
TOTAL	**2,200**	**264**	**44**	**187**

Now, how does Joe figure out what's in a specific food? That's where your nifty macrocounter comes into play. From MyFitnessPal to MyMacros, there are tons of apps out there. They'll give him the exact breakdown on just about everything he eats. And like that, Joe has the leeway to construct a diet that fits him best, as long as if fits within his macros and calories for his goal.

It has gotten to the point for me that I can track my macros without much effort. I know the numbers of most of the foods I eat, and I've been at it long enough that I can eyeball measurements. If I have an egg, I know already that there's seven grams of protein in it. It won't take you very long to have the same Rain Man–like skills.

Breakfast	Calories kcal	Carbs g	Fat g	Protein g
Friendly Farms – Greek Yogurt – Plain, 2 cup (227 g)	260	18	1	46
Dymatize – Elite 100% Whey Protein Cookies & Cream, 69.8 g	260	6	3	50
Taylor Organic – Baby Spinach, 15 oz. (2o.)	100	15	0	10
Eggs – Whole Egg (1 white + 1 yellow), 4 egg	280	4	20	24
Milk – Reduced fat, 2% milkfat, 1 cup	122	11	5	8
Chicken – Breast, meat only, cooked, roasted, 100g	165	0	4	31
Bananas – Raw, 86g	77	20	0	1
Millville – Bran Flakes (Correct), 43.5g	165	36	1	5
The Bakery – Soft Chocolate Chip Cookies, 4 cookie(s)	480	68	20	4
Mahatma – Thai Jasmine Rice, 485g (cooked)	795	179	0	15
TOTAL	**2,704**	**357**	**54**	**194**

Note how Joe was still able to enjoy foods he loved (like rice and cookies!) but could still create a caloric deficit by eating less of them.

These days when I walk into a grocery store, I don't see food, I see numbers. I see their macros. If I go to the butcher section, all I see are fats and proteins. If I'm in the pasta section, all I see is carbs. If I see nut butters, all I see is fat. I go to the fish section, and I'll see a piece of salmon and say to myself, "That's twenty-five grams of protein, a little bit of fat, and no carbs." In the cereal aisle, I'll say, "What's up carbs? How y'all doing?"

During my early research and experimentation with #IIFYM, I was psychotic about counting every little number—and it helped

EAT WHAT YOU WANT—EVEN POP-TARTS

a lot at first, until I figured out the right balance for Lean Life. Now I can just have fun with it.

I've found that too much obsession over any aspect of health or fitness makes you no longer enjoy it, but you need to go through the process of counting your macros to learn how to be self-sufficient. Eventually, you'll control these numbers; they won't control you. Your diet doesn't have to dictate your life.

As for how much fat you'll lose and how fast it'll happen, it varies by individual and how low you set your calories. It's important to know that fat loss isn't linear. Let's say Joe is on track to lose one pound a week. During the first week or two, he may not lose any weight, but come the fourth week, he may lose four pounds. Or he may lose two pounds the first two weeks and then nothing the next week. The whole point is that you're probably not going to lose the same amount each week, even if you're consistent with your calorie deficit. But taken over time, you'll see the significant differences. So don't get frustrated after trying this approach for a week or two and not feeling like you're progressing.

Besides, improvements shouldn't be drastically fast. The safest amount a moderately overweight person should lose is one to two pounds a week over the long term. If you're severely obese, you can lose more than that, but the best range to aim for is one to two pounds a week. Sure, you can go on a crazy crash diet, but good luck trying to keep that up in the long run. Extended extreme weight loss won't make you feel too hot and can throw your hormones out of whack. Plus, it'll only make you miserable and less likely to follow Lean Life successfully. We're talking about following the tortoise approach, here, not the hare approach. In other words, be patient. And consult with your doctor before you try any diet or exercise program.

Now a word on cardio exercise. If it's your hobby, that's great. Go run a marathon. But I'm not telling you to do it. By definition, cardio exercise is a low-intensity physical activity that raises your heart rate. It involves the movement of large muscles and generates weight loss by burning a large number of calories when performed during an extended period of time.

The most common strategy people use to lose weight is to start doing more cardio exercises. Cardio shouldn't be the staple in your training program, though, unless you really enjoy it.

Instead, focus on weight training. It's a lot better for building and maintaining your muscle mass, which will increase your metabolism. From there, cardio can be a supplementary exercise. You can try high-intensity interval training, which consists of short bursts of sprints followed by a longer rest or recovery, done about five to eight times. Or low-intensity, steady-state cardio like taking a thirty to sixty minute walk.

My favorite cardio to prescribe, though, is sex. Find someone you don't hate too much, or maybe someone you hate a little, and have a lot of sex with them. You'll burn as many as 250 calories a pop, and medical studies have shown that shagging stimulates neurogenesis and releases endorphins and other feel-good hormones. It reduces stress, keeps the body looking younger, and promotes better sleep.

Once you see the results and learn the balancing act between weight change and your calorie intake, you can tweak the system. You can increase the calories in your diet a little more and add some weight training or other form of exercise. Or have more sex. As to what food you should eat to drop the calories, again, that's up to you, as long as it fits your macros.

Don't get caught up in all of the nonsense about carb-free this and sugar-free that. There's no reason to vilify one specific macronutrient, whether it's carbs, fat, or protein. At the end of the day, it's a numbers game. You can't start losing weight, though, unless you ensure you're at a calorie deficit (burning more calories than you consume). All of this math and calorie counting and macro calculating may seem overwhelming to someone who's just starting out. But a lot of it is intuitive. For instance, an important rule is don't waste your calories on drinks. They don't fill you up and generally hold little nutritional value. Stick to water, unsweetened coffee or tea, and diet drinks. Additionally, aim for meals that are high in lean protein sources and fibrous veggies, even potatoes (as a carb source, since they're high volume and make you feel full). These small changes themselves can almost guarantee less calories in your diet without even pulling out your calculator.

Eventually, though, you'll need to calculate your maintenance calories as your northern compass point. This number isn't set in stone. It varies by your body type, metabolism, lifestyle, and exercise patterns. It takes you a while to find your sweet spot. It took a few weeks of trial and error to find mine, which is around 2,000 calories because I'm a little dude, around five feet six inches, and I weigh 145 pounds.

On the flip side, the maintenance calories for someone who's six feet four inches and weighs 220 pounds might be something like 3,000 calories. If you're one of them, I envy you. It's a lot harder for someone like me to go on a calorie deficit because it's hard to eat less than the small amount I'm already ingesting. A 3,000-calorie guy gets to eat way more food on a deficit than I can at maintenance. But like my high school history teacher Mr. Wilds used to say, "Life is unfair and then you die."

After the trial-and-error process of figuring out your maintenance calories, you simply need to eat fewer calories than that number. Then you need to decide on the specific foods you'll be eating. This is when personal preference plays the largest role. Take some time and construct several daily meal plans tailored to your macros and calories and cycle them throughout the week. Or stick to two or three meal plans that you've created that will help you maintain a routine.

The maintenance strategy I've found that works best for me comes from cooking my own meals from simple whole foods. It's cheaper and healthier than any other alternatives, and these all-natural, self-prepared foods have fewer calories than deep-fried takeout. I have an easier time tracking my macros in food I cook myself, too, because I'm measuring and adding all of the ingredients. If you're constantly eating out, it gets difficult to track macros because at a restaurant, the chef's main job is to make food really delicious. He doesn't give a shit about your macro intake, so there's a lot of extra calories hidden in butters and oils used for cooking seemingly healthy food options.

When I was in Egypt, I used to be able to call a butcher to send me premade boneless, skinless, and marinated chicken kabob skewers that he froze fresh for me. I'd thaw them and grill them right on the stovetop. It was incredibly convenient, and I ate them all the time. They were delicious, too. That was my go-to protein source. Many similar products are available at grocery stores across America. They're a little more expensive, but you're paying for that convenience. You don't have to be Thomas Keller or Chef Ramsay to cook at home. Just keep it simple.

Over time, you'll really enjoy being in the kitchen. I know I do. I like the social interaction of food and of preparing meals for other people. I have a good roommate situation now, and we group cook together. We'll grill a lot of chicken, someone will cook rice, and someone will cook veggies. It can be a lot of fun, especially when you incorporate other people in the mix. You can make such deep emotional connections with people when you prepare a meal with them and when you're surrounded by the smells and the sounds and the tastes. You're also showing the opposite sex that you know how things work in the kitchen, which adds up to many bonus points in the future. It's such a wonderful experience. Besides, what's the fun in going to an overpriced, loud restaurant? That's overrated in this day and age.

If you're not great in the kitchen, there are start-up companies on the Internet, such as Blue Apron, that will send a box of food to your door with directions on how to prep it, cook it, and turn it into a gourmet meal. That's always an option.

While most of the IIFYM crew that I follow online are big on home-cooked meals, there are oddballs who always eat frozen pizzas and go to In-N-Out Burger. For example, Kane Sumabat is one. If you look at his Instagram, all you'll see is green tea, ice cream, frozen pizzas, and burgers. What you don't see is his crazy discipline and determination, which he's had for twenty-plus years, and the guy's physique speaks for itself. If there's one physical example of somebody who epitomizes IIFYM, he comes to mind. This is his personal choice in what works for him. Is this a way to go about it if you're a complete newbie to tracking macros? Probably not.

On the other hand, I know people who make a list of the specific foods they like to eat, then use MyFitnessPal to create a set menu for the entire week in advance. By doing this, they can plan out their exact macro numbers without having to think or worry about it later. Down the line, they can repeat a day without having to make any calculations because the macros and calories are already precounted. The options are endless and really depend on your personal preference.

Most people who are new will want to start with baby steps. First focus on cutting out high-calorie drinks, juices, and almost anything that ends with -acchino from Starbucks. Second, aim for getting more protein in your diet (the goal is around one gram per pound of your goal body weight). If you do decide to follow Lean Life, I welcome you. Now get a scale and a calorie-counting app like MyFitnessPal. The scale doesn't need to be big, just one of those pocket-sized digital versions that goes for about $12 on Amazon. Funny aside: I had a friend in Egypt who wouldn't let me carry around the scale because he was afraid that if we got pulled over, the police would think I was dealing drugs.

These scales are incredibly precise, down to the 0.1 gram. Once you measure the weight of a piece of chicken, or a banana, or a half cup of peanuts, or whatever, plug the measurement into an app like MyFitnessPal and it will automatically break down the macros and calories. With any processed foods, you just need to scan its barcode with your smartphone, and the app will upload the nutritional information for you.

After a while, you won't even need the scale and the app very much. I don't micromanage my diet anymore, I just make sure I get a good amount of protein in it and don't go overboard with calories. Really, it doesn't take you long to get the hang of the macrotracking system. Once you do, you'll find that balance on the bike.

You'll start to dissect your meals with your new macro Matrix sixth sense in no time. For example, when you're making a turkey sandwich, you'll be able to say, "OK, each slice has five grams of protein. The two slices of bread are forty grams of carbs. One slice of cheese: that's nine grams of fat. Boom!" And like that, you'll have mastered the nutrition part of getting fit and trim, and that's 80 percent of the equation.

This process should be fun. Just have patience and trust it. Think about the big picture. I see a lot of people focusing too heavily on that 20 percent of balancing the bike, which is the training. They'll keep hiring personal trainers and signing up for fitness boot camps, but completely neglect the 80 percent, which is their diet. They'll just blindly throw money at the problem. (How do you think supplement companies are so profitable?) As they're concentrating solely on the pedaling, you can savor the moment as you race past them. You'll have the dedication and the discipline in your diet. You'll have the balance—minus my uncle's Pringles and Pepsi, and the skinned knees. There's a lot of online support you can get. For some people, I would recommend having a coach or someone who can hold you accountable. For more information on that, visit my website.

Takeaways

Calculate your maintenance calories, which is the number of calories you can include in your daily diet to maintain your current weight. From there, you can calculate your ideal macro intake and adjust your meal planning accordingly.

For initially counting your macros, you'll need a food scale, and an app such as MyFitnessPal to help you track the numbers in what you're eating.

Have patience. Losing body fat isn't a linear process. It takes time if done effectively.

Have fun.

Intermittent Fasting

The best of all medicines is resting and fasting.
—Benjamin Franklin

THE NOTION OF FASTING for better health and fitness goes back thousands of years. Plato fasted, saying it kept him sharper in mind and body. So did Socrates and Aristotle. In the simplest terms, to fast means to abstain from food or drink—or both—for an extended period of time. Swiss-German physician Philippus Paracelsus, one of the founding fathers of Western medicine, who lived five centuries ago, said, "Fasting is the greatest remedy—the physician within."

Spiritually, fasting means a lot more and is practiced in some form by nearly every faith. Its religious motivations are rooted in discipline and self-control, and in bringing people closer to purity and enlightenment. Plus, there's something to be said for group suffering and sacrifice for a greater cause, which religions are always so eager to encourage.

Buddhist monks don't eat after noon each day. In the Catholic,

Anglican, and Eastern Orthodox churches, Lent is a forty-day period of fasting. Mormons are encouraged to skip two consecutive meals on the first Sunday of every month and give the money they save on food to charity. Muslims fast during the holy month of Ramadan, refraining from food and liquids during daylight hours to cleanse the soul and repent.

Growing up, there weren't too many Muslim Texans who lived near me. In my small town of Temple, I was one of two kids at school who fasted during Ramadan. It was interesting, because for that reason, I felt even more special during Ramadan, as if I was almost setting the example for others to see how Muslims observe it.

When the holiday would roll around, people would say, "Oh, Mo, you're Muslim?" Then the pressure was on. I had no choice but to fast. I didn't want anyone to catch me cheating. Because the fast was from sunrise to sunset, my mom, dad, sisters, and I would wake up a little bit earlier than dawn and eat a big breakfast. We'd also host potlucks with other families so that it felt like a community thing—a big bond we all shared.

When I was in Egypt, I discovered how Ramadan can be a wonderful community experience. Over there, everyone invites people to their home to break the fast and enjoy it together. Even restaurants get involved. Chili's has a Ramadan buffet, for instance.

I certainly didn't appreciate the whole act of fasting as a kid. Most of the time, I just thought, *I'm hungry. I'm thirsty.*

The hardest part for me was the liquids. It's easy to get dehydrated in Texas. Being on the tennis team in high school during Ramadan was really tough. During tournaments when I was fasting, I'd grab a sandwich as soon as the sun went down and stuff it into my face between matches. I was a pretty good tennis player, and when I won during Ramadan, I have to admit, it gave me a feeling of self-empowerment because of the added challenge.

I'd say to myself, "Yes, I conquered!" It was my moment. I couldn't say, "Fuck yes, I conquered," because during Ramadan you're also supposed to refrain from sinful behavior like insulting and cursing. Maybe don't read this during Ramadan because I say fuck too many times.

There were many professional athletes I looked up to who inspired me. They fasted during Ramadan during crucial games or events. People like basketball star Hakeem Olajuwon, who played for the Houston Rockets when I was a kid, and Kareem Abdul-Jabbar, who I had read won NBA championships while fasting.

My own personal history with abstaining from food for extended periods of time—and the overall history of it—came very clearly to mind when I first discovered the concept of Intermittent Fasting on the Internet. My research led me to a guy named Martin Berkhan (leangains.com, Twitter handle @martinberkhan) who was the self-proclaimed Khan of Intermittent Fasting. Through his experimentation, he created one of the ultimate hacks in putting on muscle mass and staying very lean with Intermittent Fasting as the key.

I highly recommend his blog, where you can see the amazing results his clients have gotten. One of the most popular sections of his blog falls under the link "Top Ten Fasting Myths Debunked." Navigate around the site, and you'll find a goldmine of information. It's what led me down the road of experimentation and further research, where I found other fasting plans like the Alternate-Day Fast, which consists of alternating between a day of fasting and a day of eating normally, and the Warrior Diet, which promotes fasting for 20 hours and leaving open only a four-hour eating window.

The basic science behind Intermittent Fasting—in any form—is that by decreasing your eating window, you're eating less food but you're given the illusion that it's more because it's concentrated into a smaller time frame. Again, the primary reason why it—or any eating plan, for that matter—works at reducing weight is that it restricts calorie intake. Period. Yes there are many other benefits, and we'll discuss them. But from a practical standpoint, this is why it works so well. By abstaining from eating for an extended period of time, your body's glycogen stores become depleted, and you start burning stored fat. Fasting was so incredibly simple, I found, and something I had been doing for most of my life.

Studies have shown that fasting even five days a month improves your health and lowers risks to chronic ailments like heart disease and diabetes. Researchers at the University of Southern California found that mice, when given an eating cycle that included a fast for two four-day spans a month, lived longer, shed fat, were 45 percent less likely to contract cancer, had 40 percent lower blood sugar, and performed better on mental acuity tests. This is awesome news, of course, if you're a mouse looking to get smarter and lose weight. However, these studies weren't done on humans, and the research isn't completely conclusive.

It's believed that Intermittent Fasting helps the body repair itself faster by reducing inflammation and helping remove damaged cells, which improves your overall health. And test results indicate that it increases growth hormone levels in the body nearly sixfold—boosting energy, increasing muscle mass, improving healing, and slowing the aging process. Celebrities, bodybuilders, fitness models, and professional athletes pay thousands of dollars on the black market to get it in a vial, and you can maximize it in this simple process.

Many scientists and proponents of Intermittent Fasting theorize that through evolution, the human body was built to undergo extended periods without food. Think of it logically for a second: For ancient hunter-gatherers, eating was truly a feast-or-famine proposition. They would spend long stretches of time stalking a kill, often living on less than five calories a day. For this reason, it's very possible that the body is built to be most in tune with its surroundings, and poised to perform at its highest physical level, on an empty stomach. That's also probably why the body produces more adrenaline in this state to give you that burst of energy that you need to hunt.

I know that in my case, I'm more alert and more focused during the day thanks to Intermittent Fasting, and my blood sugar isn't always shooting up and down, so I feel more level-headed. When I do get hungry, I curb it with a cup of coffee or sparking water. Topo Chico is my favorite. From my personal experience, it's kind of a relief to fast during the day and keep off the snacks altogether.

Even when I look back at the month of Ramadan, I realize now that no one in my family would gain weight, even though we used to gorge ourselves with huge meals and crazy desserts late at night. I've begun to realize that maybe the Muslim traditions were based as much upon nutrition and science—that an occasional fasted state is better for you—as they were upon religion.

During my initial tries at Intermittent Fasting, my religious background was what reassured me that I could sustain the program as a long-term part of my health and fitness plan. I thought, *Oh, it's like Ramadan, without the most challenging part: abstaining from liquids.*

It took a few weeks for me to get a routine down, but when I did, I found that my life had become much simpler because I was reducing the time spent each day on meals and putting it to productive use in other ways—from working to working out. You'll see a difference, too, when you try it. Combining Intermittent Fasting with counting your macros creates a potent one-two punch for weight loss, even if you don't want to set foot in a gym. Within months, I was the leanest, body fat–wise, I had ever been in my life, and, most importantly, I kept lean.

What surprised me most about Intermittent Fasting was that I just didn't have enough time during my eight hours to eat more than my roughly 2,000 maintenance calories. It works so well that you're likely to undereat than overeat. I once read that Hugh Jackman, when he's training for his Wolverine roles, works out all day and intermittently fasts—eating 6,000 calories during his eight-hour window—to stay as lean as possible. It seems almost impossible to eat enough food and take enough supplements to consume that many calories, but he does it, somehow.

Don't worry: you don't need to be Wolverine to follow the same kind of program. If you're a CPA, a lawyer, a plumber, or a doctor and you're saying, "Well, I'd love to do that, but I work so much and I feel tired during the day," I get it. But my response is simple: this is mostly a mental barrier for you. I've worked with people all across the grid, from surgeons to accountants to teachers, and all of them have structured days and high-stress jobs. Yet it's worked for them.

Really, fasting is a matter of discipline. One of my recent personal training clients was in the military but had just been put into a more sedentary job and had gotten somewhat out of shape. He Skyped me and we spent a long time setting up his macros and getting him squared away on MyFitnessPal. A few weeks later, he e-mailed me a picture of himself. He had lost tons of weight. He was being disciplined with his diet, but not too strict. He'd sneak in the occasional Ben and Jerry's here and there, but that was fine. He also gained a lot of strength and had progressed on all of his lifts. He told me how much he enjoyed the process and how his lifestyle had improved.

I've found that the most challenging part of Intermittent Fasting isn't sticking with the program; it's just getting started. It takes a couple of weeks for your body to adjust to the eating cycle and to rearrange your lifestyle to fit your time and preferences. It's a dance at first. I went through it too. You're figuring out the body language and moves of your partner and how you can move in sync. By the third or fourth week, though, most people have it perfected.

What's most encouraging about the early stages are the results you'll likely see after the first six weeks. If during the first week or two there isn't that big of a difference, don't be discouraged. Keep at it. The progress over time, though, is what gives you the motivation to keep going. The body changes are noticeable in the mirror. You'll say, "Look at me, I'm leaner!" And you'll want to keep the momentum going. I know that in my first couple of months, I slimmed down at a pace that I wouldn't have wanted to maintain long term, for health reasons, but in the early stages it was fine. So once you start the program, keep at it, enjoy the difference it makes in your appearance, and trust the process.

Of course, I can't emphasize enough that before you start Intermittent Fasting, or any nutrition or fitness program, you should consult with your physician. You could have underlying health issues that would put you at risk. The whole point of this book is to help you live a healthier life, not to place you in danger for the sake of looking better. You need to be smart and responsible.

If you want to get the most out of your workouts, I recommend you lift weights in a fasted state while your insulin sensitivity is high and your body is in full fat-burning mode. Personally, it's what I do. I prefer to get a majority of my calories post-workout and take advantage of my body's insulin sensitivity (insulin is highly anabolic) in this state. I also don't want blood being sidetracked to my digestive system when I'm at the gym.

When I was a kid, and later when I was living in Egypt, I was obsessed with that meal before working out—planning it and then waiting a few hours before heading to the gym. I thought I needed to wait for the food to digest so that I would have energy, but digestion can take up to ten hours, so your body is still digesting food from yesterday if you work out in the morning. It's not like putting coal in a furnace. During this long lag, I sometimes got sidetracked and didn't get around to exercising. It all just became too much of a commitment, a chore. I don't have to deal with any of that now, since I work out when fasting. Two-thirds of the day is open to me for exercise. And when I'm working out now, I feel really pumped.

I should add a note about breakfast here. You've always heard that it's the most important meal of the day. But if you're fasting for eight hours when you sleep, and during the four hours before and after bed, you're not going to be eating that early morning meal. The concept behind a healthy breakfast, from a nutritional standpoint, is that it keeps you satisfied for much of the morning, so you won't feel like snacking on thirteen donuts in the break room at work later. In turn, you'll be healthier. This reasoning is irrelevant when Intermittent Fasting.

I, for one, love breakfast foods. Turkey bacon and eggs are so full of protein. I eat lots of oatmeal and even pancakes. I've told you about my connection to Pop-Tarts. But since food is just a bunch of numbers to me now, I don't feel bound to just eating them first thing in the morning. Who cares if I eat them in the afternoon?

What you'll find when you're Intermittent Fasting, though, is that you generally only feel like eating one big protein meal during the day—whether it's all breakfast foods or steak, chicken or fish. I usually combine it with a lot of fibrous vegetables—for the carbs, which we're not cutting, remember. In this way, the food takes a bit longer to digest, and I'm still at a calorie deficit without feeling hungry. What you'll find when you're Intermittent Fasting is that you'll feel full from less food because you just get full a lot faster. By saving up your calories for the day and having two larger meals of mostly protein, veggies (fibrous veggies), and carbs such as potatoes and rice, you'll stay full and the food will take eight-plus hours to digest.

When I was still studying in Cairo and first established my Intermittent Fasting routine, it was seriously one of the best moments of my life. I felt like I was finally rid of the shackles of meal planning and could better focus my energy on my medical school studies, comedy performances, and social life. It was so debilitating for me to be overweight. I was so self-conscious. I was afraid that patients wouldn't take me seriously if they thought I couldn't even look after my own health and fitness. I was ashamed that I wasn't setting a better example. I thought, *How can I tell patients with diabetes that they need to change their lifestyle, lose weight, make sacrifices, improve their diet if I can't follow my own advice?*

Have you ever seen the trainers on the TV show *The Biggest Loser*? They're ripped. Are any of them going to be overweight? It would be preposterous. At the low point of my fitness journey in Egypt, I felt the same way about my out-of-shape self. Preposterous.

Now I feel better about myself emotionally as well as physically. I have a better self-image, but my positive emotions are more rooted in biology. My body is working more like the machine nature intended it to be, and my eating habits are never out of whack anymore, resulting in a better sense of overall well-being. And to think the secret to this success is fasting—something I'd already been doing for Ramadan my whole life.

Takeaways
- Fasting is a tradition deeply rooted in all human societies.
- There are a number of potential health benefits connected to fasting, including anti-aging properties and higher mental acuity.
- Intermittent Fasting is the act of setting aside a certain number of hours daily when you refrain from eating and drink only noncalorie beverages. The usual number is 16 hours of fasting, leaving you with an eight-hour eating window.
- Intermittent Fasting helps you lose weight because your body shifts into fat-burning mode after an extended period of not eating, and it also partly restricts your calorie intake because you have less time and opportunity to snack on junk.

5

Reverse Pyramid Weight Training: Spend Less Time with Sociopaths!

> *Our bodies are our gardens—our will are our gardeners.*
> –William Shakespeare

IN HIS BOOK *The Tipping Point*, Malcolm Gladwell writes about how the quick, easy solutions are often the best ones, even though we tend to overlook them. He uses the Band-Aid as an example. The little sticky piece of plastic with gauze glued to it has helped billions of people keep moving in their daily lives when they would otherwise be forced to stop and waste time finding another, more involved solution to stop a cut from bleeding. Yet somehow we look at "Band-Aid" solutions as being not ideal ones.

This attitude doesn't make sense. Why do we want to make things more complicated? Why should we look reflexively at the simple answers with suspicion? The "Band-Aid solution" to a problem is actually the best possible kind you can find, "because it involves solving a problem with the minimum amount of effort and time and cost," he writes. Yet it works really, really well.

The problem, according to Gladwell, is that humans are hardwired to "disdain" easy answers. We feel like we need to earn the right solution through lots and lots of effort, sweat, and sacrifice. Like the best results are supposed to be really complicated. So we ignore the "convenient shortcut," and the "way to make a lot out of a little." We ignore efficiency. There's also money in complication. A lot of people in the fitness and health industries go out of their way to make a very simple system complex so that the consumer has to pay for help to understand it. They don't want you to be able to function independently.

You may be suspicious about the idea that you can spend less time worrying about eating, put less effort into preparing meals, and spend less time in the gym yet still lose weight and get fitter and stronger. Believing that things like this are possible goes against our hard wiring. I'm telling you, though, let go of your suspicions. With Lean Life, the best solution really is the least complicated one!

After all, efficiency is defined in the dictionary as "the ratio of useful work performed compared to the total energy expended." In other words, it means making a lot out of a little. That's also the perfect definition for Lean Life. It's the convenient shortcut. It's like Gladwell's Band-Aid!

The most time-effective portion of Lean Life is the very quick weight-lifting session. If you're a beginner to the weight room, three days of total body workouts will be enough. If you have more experience, add three days of push/pull exercises and legs. If you want maximum efficiency while gaining strength, then Reverse Pyramid training will be the most efficient way to achieve it.

You'll discover that you can spend as little as ninety minutes a week in the gym and still see incredible results. I've already described how the benefits to weight training is building muscle, which in turn increases your metabolism and lets you build a very good-looking physique once you shed the fat. In the process, you'll avoid the dreaded skinny-fat, no-definition look that a lot of people fall into after losing weight. During your fat-loss journey, you'll simultaneously be building muscle on your frame.

Imagine a sculptor shaving down a block of marble. Right now you and your love handles, or saddlebags, are that block of marble. And you want to sculpt yourself down to look like a Greek god or goddess. For that to happen, you have to build muscle mass. Strong is the new skinny. No one just wants to be skinny anymore; they want to be muscular too. Efficient weight training is the way to do it.

You might not have ever heard of Reverse Pyramid weight training before. It's a bit unconventional, because it's more intense but less time consuming. The concept behind it is that you're able to get in and out of the gym faster, while gaining maximum strength benefits. People can be skeptical of it at first, because—as I've said—we all have a natural disdain for easy answers. I'll give you an example.

I went to a gym in my hometown of Temple, Texas, recently and ran into a friend from high school who I hadn't seen in a few years. He saw that my body had changed completely. I was leaner and stronger than he had ever seen me, but he had stayed the same. Even though he still worked out regularly, he wasn't seeing the progress he wanted to see anymore.

He saw me bench-pressing 225 pounds, and said, "Wow, dude, I want to be able to do that!"

I told him he could and described the Reverse Pyramid method. His response, "There's no way that will work for me."

He didn't think there was any such thing as a simple answer. That "no way" attitude is the first hurdle everyone has to clear when starting Reverse Pyramid training. Not that everyone is ready for such a high-intensity workout at the start.

If you're a beginner I'd recommend a more conventional workout split such as the one that follows. It's a super simple, three-times-a-week, full-body program that focuses on compound movements and engages the total body. Feel free to use machines if you aren't experienced with barbells or dumbbells.

Beginner Workout Table

MONDAY
Overhead press
3 sets x 12 reps
Bench press
3 sets x 12 reps
Lat pull down
3 sets x 12 reps
Back-supported row
3 sets x 12 reps
Leg press
3 sets x 12 reps

TUESDAY
30-minute walk

WEDNESDAY
Overhead press
3 sets x 12 reps
Bench press
3 sets x 12 reps
Lat pull down
3 sets x 12 reps
Seated-supported row
3 sets x 12 reps
Leg press
3 sets x 12 reps

THURSDAY
30-minute walk

FRIDAY
Overhead press
3 sets x 12 reps
Bench press
3 sets x 12 reps
Lat pull down
3 sets x 12 reps
Supported row
3 sets x 12 reps
Leg press
3 sets x 12 reps

SATURDAY
Rest

SUNDAY
Rest

REVERSE PYRAMID WEIGHT TRAINING

For somebody a little bit more advanced, we can add a little more volume and split your workout into push, pull, and legs, also three times a week, with no more than four or five exercises per session. Here's an example:

MONDAY
Push
Overhead press
4 sets x 12 reps
Incline bench press
4 sets x 12 reps
Bench press
4 sets x 12 reps
Triceps extension
4 sets x 12 reps

TUESDAY
30-minute walk

WEDNESDAY
Pull
Lat pull down
4 sets x 12 reps
Close-grip reverse pull down
4 sets x 12 reps
Supported row
4 sets x 12 reps
Bicep barbell curl
4 sets x 12 reps

THURSDAY
30-minute walk

FRIDAY
Legs
Leg press
4 sets x 12 reps
Leg extensions
4 sets x 12 reps
Leg curl
4 sets x 12 reps
Calve raises
4 sets x 12 reps

SATURDAY
Rest

SUNDAY
Rest

Now if you're somebody like me—or my high school friend in the gym that day—who wants the biggest bang for your buck when it comes to gaining strength and spending the least amount of time in the gym, you should probably try Reverse Pyramid training. My friend insisted he couldn't do it, so I told him, "Not only can you do it, but you're going to try it right now."

I spotted him and he did two bench press reps, nearly maximum weight. He was shaking and it was really hard for him. He told me afterward, "Oh, that was really painful."

"That's the point," I said. "You're supposed to be challenged. That's how muscle grows!"

And like that, he was hooked. Reverse Pyramid is intense, but with intensity comes added strength and muscle mass. Instead of focusing on volume and increasing sets and reps, you're now concentrating on making progress with weight. Unlike with the long, slow burn of a typical workout, you're wasting no time in pushing yourself to the limit. This is not an aerobic exercise. You're in a "weight" room and you're "weight" training, after all. With this workout, you're not sitting around the gym exposed to the company of muscle-head psychopaths either; you're in and out as quickly as possible. (With that being said, I still do love the Zen of weight training in a gym.)

The theory behind Reverse Pyramid training is that by starting with the heaviest weights first, you have the ability to put your muscles to the absolute max before they fatigue. By doing this, you're creating a stimulus that causes your muscles to grow. Increasing weight takes a mental commitment, but it's the most efficient weight-training protocol if you can get over that intimidation barrier.

With Reverse Pyramid, you're not using any new core lifts or techniques. They're the same as with the other exercises I've recommended here. It's just the numbers and weights that are different. With Reverse Pyramid, you start with the heaviest weight for six to eight reps for the first set. You rest for two to three minutes and perform the second set with 10 percent less weight. And that's it. Just two sets! Now, those six to eight reps are brutal. The weight should be heavy enough that you can't do even a single extra rep. If you find yourself able to do more, then the weight should be heavier. It goes without saying—though I'll say it anyway—you should use proper form, and have a spotter, whenever you're doing Reverse Pyramid. If you can't find a spotter, stick to machines. Again, remember that fasting and macro counting are 80 percent of balancing that bike, and only 20 percent is the weight training.

Almost as important as the physical benefits of Reverse Pyramid training are the psychological ones. If you notice, even with the beginner and intermediate plans, without incorporating Reverse Pyramid, you're still only in the gym three days a week. This helps psychologically because your schedule is freer. Traditional programs that advise going to the gym nearly every day make weight training feel like a job, and it quickly becomes monotonous and boring. Sometimes a break is justifiably needed though. Besides, as they say, absence makes the heart grow fonder. A relatable real-life example would be going to family events. It's great to see everybody you know and uncle Jim for an occasional meal or birthday party, but the key to keeping the love is doing it in limited doses.

I know that when I first started limiting my weight-training sessions to three days a week when I was in medical school in Cairo, it definitely revived the fun of going to the gym—and looking in the mirror—for me. That combined with Intermittent Fasting and tracking macros created crazy progress that I had never seen before. I was blown away by the results and how much sense tying together the science on these three concepts made. The simple solutions really were the most elegant and effective ones, even though my inner self kept yelling, "This isn't possible! Success can't come this easily! It's got to be more complicated, more painful."

I had lost weight so quickly, that my body image hadn't had time to catch up. I still considered myself overweight and felt like I needed to shave off more pounds. But my friends kept saying, "You're batshit crazy! If you lose any more weight, you'll disappear!" Eventually, I came to my senses.

All the while, I was getting stronger, leaner, and spending less time at the gym, while the people around me were doing the same thirty-six sets of shoulder exercises, thinking they're going to be the next Mr. Olympia but getting nowhere.

When people see something new and innovative, whether it's an app that gets you a ride somewhere for cheaper than taking a cab, or a computer watch, or a new workout program, they want to find out more about it and try it. As long as they don't think it's a "Band-Aid approach." I know that when I'm at the gym and I see someone doing a new exercise—and doing it well—I'll ask the person about it. I might be able to gain some knowledge, or some new understanding. This curiosity is what led me down the path to Lean Life in the first place and the brought me the results I've achieved.

Hopefully, you see that the strategies and lessons I've outlined here will spare you the thirteen years' learning curve that I went through and that they will give you the tools to get you in the best shape of your life. To succeed, you're going to need to make that leap of self-confidence by saying, "I'm going to lift." Or, "I'm going to stay disciplined with my macro limits." Or, "I'm not going to break my fast." And fall in love with the journey. Happiness lies in the process itself.

With almost every journey I've taken in life, I've usually thought that when I reached the final destination, I'd be happier. In medical school, I thought, *Wow, this is stressful*, but looking back now, I had some of the best times of my life during that period. I just didn't realize it at the time. The journey was fun, but I didn't stop to appreciate it. I didn't give myself permission to be happy.

I've noticed that a lot of my fellow comedians need to seek validation from others. They think, *If the audience thinks this joke is funny, I'll feel better about myself*. But at the end of the day it's your own responsibility to feel good about yourself. While having a college or medical degree, or being funny on stage, or having a great physique are all great accomplishments, you don't need to reach those goals to be happy. Enjoy the sights, sounds, and tastes of getting there and be proud of your commitment and progress.

The fun part with Lean Life comes when you begin to trust your body, and the program, and your ability to achieve great results. You'll start tracking the increase in weights, and your progression in strength, with anticipation. You won't want to miss a workout session, and even when you're tired and sapped of energy from work or just the slings and arrows of life, you'll still somehow muster that inner strength to lift that weight and finish that last rep. You'll find yourself filled with that rare and exciting feeling of genuine pride.

Takeaways

- Sometimes the simplest solutions truly are the best ones. This rule also applies to weight training.
- Beginners should stick to a more conventional three-times-a-week, full-body program.
- Intermediates can add volume and split workouts into push, pull, and legs, also three times a week.
- People who are more advanced in the weight room can try Reverse Pyramid training.
- With Reverse Pyramid, you lift the heaviest weights in the first set, pushing your muscles to the limit and stimulating strength and growth.
- Reverse Pyramid consists of just two sets of six to eight reps, two minutes apart. That's it. Fast and efficient.

Lean Life

Every patient carries her or his own doctor inside.
—Albert Schweitzer

THERE'S AN OLD CHINESE SAYING that goes, "Teachers open the door; you enter by yourself." In describing to you my personal journey over the past thirteen years with fitness and nutrition, outlining the basics of Lean Life, and becoming a doctor, I've tried to open the door for you in this book. But you can only enter by yourself. I want you to know that at the end of the day, there's only so much that a health professional can do about your health and welfare. The rest is completely up to you.

I decreased my body fat, increased my strength, and improved my mental and physical health through very simple, efficient steps involving Intermittent Fasting, flexible dieting, and weight training. Beyond these measurements, though, the Lean Life system has empowered me. It has made me realize that I'm in charge of my body and my life.

I hope you learned the same lessons. Your life and

circumstances are unique. You don't need to follow cookie-cutter advice or cookie-cutter plans that were spit out by the evil fitness industry. Lean Life is something different—something meant to last forever.

Whether you choose to use just the suggestions on fasting, weight training, or flexible dieting, it's up to you. Maybe you want to cherry-pick ideas. Or try all three. It's completely up to you. These concepts are intended to cut through all of the noise when it comes to fitness and nutrition advice. I know that because there's so much money to be made by the fitness industry in complicating the process, many of us suffer from analysis paralysis and don't know whom to trust. I'm just trying to save you time and effort, and make things more efficient for you, just like Lean Life itself. All you have to do is unleash the doctor within and take responsibility for your own health.

Lastly, it's important that I mention the following people who were vital to my research. They are the pioneers, I believe, in taking the fitness and personal health industry forward and out of the hands of corporations. They put a wealth of content out there that's available to the public, and they lend their time and expertise to others out of an amazing generosity of spirit. I was able to apply their teachings in creating Lean Life. Please check them out.

Kane Sumabat (Instagram handle: @timbawolffff)
IIFYM extraordinaire. Someone I truly admire, and he has so much passion for the art of bodybuilding.

Martin Berkhan (Instagram handle: @martinberkhan)
A badass nutritional consultant who completely shat on how we used to look at dieting protocols.

Alberto Nunez (Instagram handle: nunez3dmj)
He's a lifetime drug-free bodybuilder, nutrition guru, and fitness coach with a strength-training company called 3D Muscle Journey (3dmusclejourney.com).

Layne Norton, PhD (Instagram handle: @biolayne)
He's a competitive bodybuilder who has a huge following and posts a lot of free content on weight training.

Tony "TBone" Somera (Instagram handle: @supersaiyantbone)
He's an expert macro counter and fitness freak, and a very generous person with his time. He doesn't have a huge following but is extremely knowledgeable.

Alan Aragon (Website: alanaragon.com)
He's a nutrition advisor and leader in cutting through the bullshit put out by the corporate fitness industry. Aragon gives scientific, evidence-based information for the health and fitness movement.

Lyle McDonald (Website: bodyrecomposition.com)
He's a consultant who helps people change their bodies by using science-based approaches to fitness, fat loss, nutrition, and muscle-mass gain.

Brad Pilon (Website: bradpilon.com)
He is one of the leading experts on Intermittent Fasting and author of the book *Eat Stop Eat*. He blogs constantly and shares all sorts of advice and information.

The online community is a limitless resource where you can share and learn from others. You can even connect with me! My handle is drmofitness (on Facebook, Twitter, Instagram, and Snapchat). I'm looking forward to hearing about your success.

www.ingramcontent.com/pod-product-compliance
Lightning Source LLC
Chambersburg PA
CBHW031158020426
42333CB00013B/728